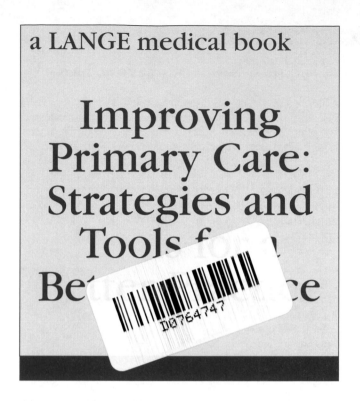

a LANGE medical book

Improving Primary Care: Strategies and Tools for a Better Practice

Thomas Bodenheimer, MD, MPH
Center for Excellence in Primary Care
Department of Family and Community Medicine
University of California, San Francisco

Kevin Grumbach, MD
Center for Excellence in Primary Care
Professor and Chair
Department of Family and Community Medicine
University of California, San Francisco

Lange Medical Books/McGraw-Hill
Medical Publishing Division

*New York Chicago San Francisco Lisbon London Madrid
Mexico City Milan New Delhi San Juan Seoul
Singapore Sydney Toronto*

The **McGraw·Hill** Companies

Improving Primary Care: Strategies and Tools for a Better Practice

2 3 4 5 6 7 8 9 0   DOC/DOC   0 9 8 7

ISBN 13: 978-0-07-144738-6
ISBN 10: 0-07-144738-5

This book was set in Times Roman by International Typesetting and Composition.
The editors were James F. Shanahan and Regina Y. Brown.
The production supervisor was Sherri Souffrance.
The cover designer was Mary McKeon.
Photo credit: Image Source/Getly Images®.
The indexer was Susan Hunter.
RR Donnelley was printer and binder.
This book is printed on acid-free paper.

Cataloging-in-Publication Data is on file for this title at the Library of Congress.

Notice

Medicine is an ever-changing science. As new research and clinical experience broaden our knowledge, changes in treatment and drug therapy are required. The authors and the publisher of this work have checked with sources believed to be reliable in their efforts to provide information that is complete and generally in accord with the standards accepted at the time of publication; however, in view of the possibility of human error or changes in medical sciences, neither the editors nor the publisher nor any other party who has been involved in the preparation or publication of this work warrants that the information contained herein is in every respect accurate or complete, and they disclaim all responsibility for any errors or omissions or for the results obtained from use of the information contained in this work. Readers are encouraged to confirm the information contained herein with other sources. For example and in particular, readers are advised to check the product information sheet included in the package of each drug they plan to administer to be certain that the information contained in this work is accurate and that changes have not been made in the recommended dose or in the contraindications for administration. This recommendation is of particular importance in connection with new or infrequently used drugs.

Contents

Preface

We wrote this book for both policy and personal reasons. Policy wise, primary care is troubled. Imagine if primary care did not exist. Could orthopedic surgeons be expected to handle all ankle sprains and low back pain? How could the few endocrinologists in each city care for the growing millions of people with diabetes? Would cardiologists trained to insert stents into coronary arteries have the time or interest to control the blood pressures of 20 million people with hypertension?

Yet the history of health care in the United States, reinforced by recent developments, has relegated primary care to second-class status, causing students to seek non–primary care careers, creating stress and frustration among primary care practitioners, leaving many primary care practices financially unstable, and forcing patients to wait several weeks for a rushed 15-minute appointment. Primary care physicians are being asked to do far more than they can.

At the same time, new ideas abound in the primary care enterprise. Patients are seen as partners, participating in decisions while taking more responsibility for their health. Primary care innovators are advancing new models to guide improvement in primary care practices. The computer revolution, in tandem with other innovations, has the potential to facilitate information exchange among caregivers and between caregivers and patients—altering the entire flow of the workday.

To raise the spirits of primary care and to institutionalize innovation—from large integrated systems to one-doctor offices—primary care needs far more support from the power centers of medicine and society. As an acknowledgement of the huge increase in clinical responsibilities borne by its practitioners, primary care deserves more reimbursement. Primary care merits media recognition, receiving as much airtime as face transplants and genetic modifications.

On a personal level, primary care has dominated our lives. Between the two of us, we have spent over 50 years working as primary care physicians— in private practice, community health centers, and public hospital clinics. We have had unforgettably wonderful experiences, involving patients whose lives became intertwined with ours. We have also endured the chaos of the typical primary care day, when an elderly man with chest pain or a young woman contemplating suicide takes priority, and pushes aside all other activities. Repeatedly, we have had to tell patients, worried that they might have cancer, that the first radiology appointment we were able to arrange was 6 weeks away. We have told people to come on time at 2 P.M. and we have not seen them until 3:30 P.M. We have given patients complicated medication regimens and, with only a few minutes available, have failed to explain clearly what the patients were supposed to do. We learned Spanish and then found many of our new patients monolingual in Cantonese. With our colleagues—clinicians, nurses, health educators, medical assistants, receptionists, and specialists—we have experienced mutual respect, lived through hours of stress, and enjoyed times of fun.

Whether experiencing the joy of helping a patient over an illness, or feeling the pain of helplessly watching someone inexorably slide downhill, primary care is always intense.

This book's opening chapter recounts the importance of primary care, its problems, and the crisis it faces. The second chapter looks to the future, exploring the vision of twenty-first century primary care. Chapters 3 through 10 provide detailed accounts of the innovations required to bring this vision into reality. The final chapter and the brief conclusion turn from the primary care microsystem to the health care macrosystem, focusing on the inequities of primary care reimbursement. To rejuvenate primary care, innovation is needed at both the micro- and the macrosystem levels.

We hope this book will provide some ideas on how to provide better care for patients while increasing the satisfaction and reducing the frustration of primary care practice. When we started practicing primary care years ago, we would have appreciated having this book to assist us in our journey.

Acknowledgments

Primary care includes family physicians, general internists, general pediatricians, nurse practitioners, and physician assistants. Because the difficulties of primary care are more acute for adult primary care, we have paid little specific attention to pediatrics. Hopefully, pediatricians will find the book to be helpful, particularly the chapters on the management of chronic illness and improving timely access to appointments.

The book does not address the important issues of health disparities, cultural competence, and limited health literacy in a major way. For an in-depth examination of these topics, we recommend a companion book: King T, Wheeler M, Bindman A, et al (eds.): *Medical Management of Vulnerable and Underserved Patients: Principles, Practice, and Populations*. New York, McGraw-Hill, 2006.

Portions of this book are summaries of peer-reviewed evidence, particularly for chronic care, patient self-management, and primary care teams. These reviews derive from searches of the Medline and Cochrane databases. Research on these topics generally suffers from methodologic flaws, reflecting the reality that research on quality improvement is far more difficult than trials of medications; although the quality and dose of a pill can be standardized, that is not the case for a quality improvement intervention.

Everything in life builds on the work and cooperation of others, and this book is no exception. We particularly thank Dr. Drummond Rennie, of the Journal of the American Medical Association (JAMA), who stimulated us to develop our ideas about primary care improvement. Some of this book's chapters have been adapted from articles that appeared in JAMA: 2002;288:889–893, 1775–1779, 1909–1914, 2469–2475; 2003;289: 1042–1046, 290:259–264, 2004;291:1246–1251. Copyrighted © 2002,

2003, 2004 American Medical Association. All rights reserved. Shelley Reinhardt, formerly at McGraw-Hill, encouraged us to write this book, and McGraw-Hill editor James Shanahan has become a partner in this undertaking. Our families and colleagues have accompanied us on this journey, by offering feedback or through overall support of our efforts.

Finally, we acknowledge the contributions of the hundreds of innovators who are working to improve primary care, and the tens of thousands of primary care clinicians who work long hours, with modest reward, to brighten the lives of their patients.

Thomas Bodenheimer
Kevin Grumbach
San Francisco, California
March 2006

CHAPTER ONE

The Primary Care Home

Dr. Rebecca Rushmore, a family physician, glances at her watch as she heads into the examination room to treat the last patient of the day. It is 6:15 P.M. As usual, she is running more than an hour behind schedule. She is hoping that she can arrive at her son's high school baseball game in time to see the last few innings. That hope is quickly dashed as she realizes that the patient she is about to treat is Mr. Hardaway. From years of caring for Mr. Hardaway, Dr. Rushmore knows it will be difficult to complete the visit in 10 minutes. He has poorly controlled diabetes, hypertension, and congestive heart failure complicated by depression from his recent divorce. Visits require a time-consuming review of his complicated treatment regimen and discussion of his divorce and relationship with his children. Dr. Rushmore is more conscious of the inadequacy of Mr. Hardaway's diabetic control since she started receiving periodic quality-of-care report cards from his health plan that lists him as an outlier because of his hemoglobin A1c values above 10%. Today's visit promises to be even more difficult. Mr. Hardaway's prostate-specific antigen test from 1 week ago shows an elevated level. Dr. Rushmore will need to explain the implications of the test result and suggest a referral to a urologist for prostate biopsy. Undoubtedly, he will bring up some new symptoms that he wants Dr. Rushmore to evaluate.

As Dr. Rushmore enters the examination room, she reminds herself of the satisfaction she gets from her primary care practice and of Mr. Hardaway's gratitude for the time she spends with him. But she has a sinking feeling that the days are not long enough to do all she must do for her patients and that the challenges of primary care never stop growing. She wonders whether she is either losing her stamina or trying to practice primary care in a health care world that demands drastic new approaches.

THE PRIMARY CARE HOME

Most people in the United States want a *medical home* [1]. Primary care, which addresses a majority of patients' health care needs [2], was developed to serve as the medical home.

Although some nomadic patients prefer to navigate their way through episodic encounters with emergency departments and specialty clinics, the majority benefit from and desire a primary care home. In a survey of California patients, 94% valued having a primary care physician who knew about all their medical problems. Most preferred to seek initial care for common problems from their primary care physician rather than a specialist [3].

The primary care home has several essential functions [2, 4]. Primary care offers first-contact care—a doorbell patients can ring to initiate getting help. Primary care is comprehensive—encompassing a spectrum of preventive, acute, and chronic health care needs. The primary care home is not temporary but provides longitudinal care with sustained relationships, a place where people know you. In addition, the primary care home is a base from which other accommodations–specialists and other caregivers—are arranged. Abundant evidence indicates the benefits to patients and health systems of having a primary care home with these essential attributes [2, 4].

Physicians like Dr. Rebecca Rushmore work diligently to provide a good primary care home for their patients. But more and more of Dr. Rushmore's primary care colleagues are finding that they cannot do what they are expected to do. The demands for care—that is available when patients need it, that creates interpersonal bonds between physicians and patients, and that consistently conforms to universally accepted quality guidelines—are too great, causing severe strains within primary care. Responding to these heightened demands will require a fundamental remodeling of the primary care home.

WHAT IS PRIMARY CARE?

The Institute of Medicine defines primary care as "the provision of integrated, accessible health care services by clinicians who are accountable for addressing a large majority of personal health care needs, developing a sustained partnership with patients, and practicing in the context of family and community" [2]. In her 1998 book *Primary Care: Balancing Health Needs, Services, and Technology,* Barbara Starfield, one of the world's foremost authorities on primary care, describes four pillars of primary care practice: first-contact care, continuity over time, comprehensiveness (concern for the entire patient rather than one organ system), and coordination with other parts of the health system [4]. First-contact care is the single door through which patients can enter the health care system. For patients, this means "If I get sick I can first call my primary care physician and see my primary care physician soon." Continuity signifies that patients/families have a regular source of care over a significant period of time; "Dr. Long has been my family's primary care physician for 14 years." Comprehensiveness refers to primary care's responsibility to deliver all types of health services—preventive, acute, chronic, palliative, supportive—or to arrange for such care to be provided. Patients view this attribute as "My primary care physician takes care of most of my medical problems." Coordination involves the integration of all care, no matter where or by whom the care is obtained. Patients would view coordination as "If several physicians are involved with my care, my primary care physician helps put it all together for me."

Whereas general practitioners are the primary care physicians in many nations, the United States assigns the task of primary care to several specialties—family physicians, general internists, and general pediatricians. Increasingly, primary care nurse practitioners and physician assistants are a major portion of the primary care workforce. For that reason, it is encompassing to use the term primary care clinicians (including physicians, nurse practitioners, and physician assistants) rather than primary care physicians.

WHY PRIMARY CARE?

Polly Seymour, a 55-year-old woman with private health insurance living in the United States, sees several different physicians for a variety of problems: a dermatologist for eczema, a gastroenterologist for recurrent heartburn, and an orthopedist for tendinitis in her shoulder. She may ask her gastroenterologist to treat a few general medical problems, such as borderline diabetes. On occasion, she has gone to the nearby hospital emergency room for treatment of urinary tract infections. One day Ms. Seymour feels a lump in her breast and consults a gynecologist. She is referred to a surgeon for biopsy, which indicates cancer. The surgeon performs a lumpectomy and refers her to an oncologist and radiation therapy specialist for further therapy.

Although many nations have built their health care systems on a well-established foundation of primary care, the United States, Japan, and some other nations have traditionally placed less emphasis on primary care. The experiences of patients like Polly Seymour typify the specialist-centric model of care that became dominant in the United States after World War II, with many patients consulting different specialists for different ailments, without a primary care clinician to coordinate their care. In the mid-1960s, 45% of the population had no regular physician. For 27% of those with a regular physician—that physician was a specialist [5].

Primary care physicians currently make up about 35% of the total physician supply in the United States, a number well below the 50% or more found in Canada and many European nations. Adding primary care physician assistants (44% of all physician assistants are in primary care) and primary care nurse practitioners (about 80% of all nurse practitioners) to the number of primary care physicians, primary care clinicians account for about 43% of the total U.S. clinician supply [6, 7]. Fifty-two percent of visits to doctors in 2000 were to primary care physicians [8].

Polly Seymour feels terrible. Every time she eats, she feels nauseated and frequently vomits. She has lost 8 pounds, and her oncologist is worried that her breast cancer has spread. She undergoes blood tests, an abdominal CT (Computerized Tomography) scan, and a bone scan—all of which are normal. She returns to her gastroenterologist, who tells her to stop the ibuprofen she has been taking for tendinitis. Her problem persists and the gastroenterologist performs an endoscopy, which shows mild gastric irritation. A month has passed, $5000 has been spent, and Ms. Seymour continues to vomit.

Her friend recommends a primary care physician, Dr. Steward, who takes a complete history, which reveals that she is taking tamoxifen for her breast cancer and that she began to take aspirin after stopping the ibuprofen. Dr. Steward explains that either of these medications can cause vomiting and suggests that they be stopped for a week. Ms. Seymour returns in a week, her nausea and vomiting resolved. Dr. Steward then consults the oncologist, and together they decide to restart the tamoxifen but not the aspirin. Ms. Seymour begins to feel well and gains weight while taking a reduced dose of tamoxifen. In the future, Dr. Steward handles Ms. Seymour's medical problems, referring her to specialty physicians when needed, and making sure that the advice of one consultant does not interfere with the therapy of another specialist.

While the specialist-oriented, technologically enamored U.S. health system has achieved major advances in health care, this orientation has come under criticism for contributing to high costs and inadequate quality. Advocates of a primary-care-based system have argued that patients such as Polly Seymour benefit from a more coordinated approach to their care, such as that provided by Dr. Steward. In the 1960s, the primary care movement in the United States began to achieve notable gains, culminating in the establishment of family medicine as a board-certified specialty. Encountering many subsequent challenges, primary care in the United States received a boost in the 1980s and 1990s from the advent of managed care, as most managed care plans required their enrollees to choose a primary care physician and did not allow specialist care without a referral from a primary care *gatekeeper.* Unfortunately, implementation of rigid gatekeeper rules by profit-oriented, commercial health plans engendered a public backlash against this enforced model of primary care. By the end of the twentieth century, primary care fortunes in the United States were again on the decline. However, despite the often inhospitable climate for primary care in the United States, an impressive international body of research demonstrates that a primary care-centered health system has major advantages—for patients, specialists, and the costs of health care. The central functions of primary care—first-contact care, continuity, comprehensiveness, and coordination—add value to the medical care system by improving quality and reducing cost [2, 4].

THE VALUE OF A PRIMARY CARE HOME

Primary Care and Quality

Continuity of care is more likely to be present when care is provided by generalists rather than specialists [4]. Increased continuity is associated with better outcomes for diabetic patients [9], improved control of hypertension [10], and less reliance on emergency department services [10]. A review of 40 studies found that continuity of care was almost always associated with improved clinical outcomes, including delivery of preventive care, chronic illness management indicators, and maternity care outcomes [11].

Persons whose care meets a primary care oriented model are more likely to receive recommended preventive services, to adhere to treatment, and to be satisfied with their care [12–15]. Nations with a greater primary care orientation tend to have better performance on health indicators such as infant mortality and life expectancy [16]. Within the United States, states with more primary care physicians—but not specialists—have better population health indicators such as total mortality, heart disease, and cancer mortality, and neonatal mortality [17].

Primary Care, Specialists, and the Health System

Specialists and other providers depend on a well-functioning primary care system to optimize the effectiveness of their role in the health system [18]. Primary care plays an important *filtering role* through the referral process, assuring that specialists can concentrate their efforts on patients with complex conditions requiring specialized expertise. If primary care clinicians are in short supply, patients go to specialists for their primary care needs. Cardiologists care for essential hypertension. Urologists care for upper respiratory infections. While one study found that 28% of specialists' time was spent providing primary care [19], many specialists do not appreciate doing primary care, lack primary care competencies, and lag behind primary care physicians in providing preventive care services [15, 20]. Primary care clinicians play other important roles that support the overall integrity of the health system, such as caring for patients with undifferentiated chronic symptoms that defy discrete diagnosis, and serving as an adaptive reservoir of clinicians who can flexibly take on added responsibilities in response to changing epidemiologic and health care trends, such as incorporating mental health or oral health services into primary care [18]. Specialists need primary care physicians.

Primary Care and Health Care Costs

For the health system and the overall economy, a system with underdeveloped primary care creates major cost pressures. Patients with a regular generalist physician have lower overall costs than those without [21–23]. Generalists and specialists provide comparable quality of care at lower cost for a variety of conditions such as diabetes, hypertension, and lower back pain [23–26].

Nineteen of twenty studies demonstrated that continuity of care, which is more likely when care is provided by generalists rather than specialists, is associated with reductions in hospitalizations and emergency department visits, and declines in overall costs [11].

Increased primary care to population ratios reduce hospitalization rates for six ambulatory-care-sensitive conditions in the United States [27]. Health care costs are higher in regions with higher ratios of specialist-to-generalist physicians [28].

Nations with a greater proportion of their physicians practicing primary care medicine tend to have lower per capita health expenditures than nations with a greater proportion of specialists [4]. Within the United States, great differences in per capita costs for Medicare patients exist between one metropolitan area and another, differences unexplained by demographic, socioeconomic, or burden-of-illness factors. High-cost areas tend to have a greater preponderance of specialists; yet Medicare enrollees in high-cost regions did not receive better quality of care than a demographically similar population in low-cost regions [29, 30].

In a remarkable study, Baicker and Chandra examined Medicare data by state using 24 common quality indicators. High quality was significantly associated with lower per capita Medicare expenditures. States with more specialists per capita had lower quality and higher per capita Medicare expenditures [31].

Primary Care is Evidence-Based

In summary, a health system based on primary care is associated with better quality and reduced costs. This body of research demonstrates that a primary-care-centered system constitutes evidence-based health policy. It is universally accepted that evidence-based interventions constitute the proper standard for guiding clinical practices. Given the preponderance of research on the value of primary care, shouldn't a primary-care-centered system be accepted as the evidence-based standard for organizing health care systems?

THE ENDANGERED PRIMARY CARE HOME

In the mid-1990s, primary care in the United States looked like a winner. Increasing numbers of medical students were choosing primary care careers. Rapidly-growing HMOs (Health Maintenance Organizations) based their care structure on the primary care coordinator. In 1996, 77% of Americans reported having a primary care provider [32]. In one survey, 94% of people seeing a primary care physician valued the experience [3].

By 2003, the momentum had shifted. HMOs were in decline and the primary care gatekeeper model was leaving the field [33]. Many medical students soured on primary care careers. While clinical responsibilities grew, primary care incomes declined relative to those of many specialists. Patients, while continuing to applaud the concept of the family physician, were complaining about having trouble getting a timely appointment with their primary care physician. Only one-third of adult patients in Massachusetts considered their primary care physician's knowledge about them to be excellent or good [32]. A survey of Medicare beneficiaries in 13 states found a decline in patients' satisfaction with the primary care physician-patient relationship [32]. Twenty-four percent of primary care physicians felt that the scope of care they were expected to provide was greater than what is reasonable [34].

Some experts predicted "primary care's time has finally come and gone" [35]. A prominent primary care advocate worried "Primary care in America is an endangered species" [36]. Primary care leaders in other nations, for example, the United Kingdom [37], are also concerned about their profession. In the worst possible scenario, primary care could enter a *death spiral* in which the gap widens between what primary care can provide and what the public wants, incomes of primary care physicians continue to fall relative to that of specialists, fewer medical students enter primary care, primary care is therefore even less able to fulfill the public's expectations, and the entire enterprise spirals downhill [35].

Considerable evidence supports the view that primary care is in crisis.

Primary Care Physician Dissatisfaction

Many primary care physicians are stressed, some are exhausted physically and emotionally, and almost all are overwhelmed with crammed schedules, inefficient work environments, and unrewarding administrative tasks [1]. Anecdotes of early retirement among primary care physicians are common.

Primary care physician satisfaction has fallen, though to a varying degree in different surveys. A national survey found that 38.5% of primary care physicians were very satisfied with their career in 2001 compared with 42.4% in 1997 [38]. A California physician survey found that 42% of primary care physicians were very satisfied in 2001 compared with 46% in 1996 [39]. A Kaiser Family Foundation survey performed in 2001 found that about 80% of physicians (primary care and specialty) were satisfied with their relationships with patients and professional challenges, but only 43–44% were satisfied with their professional autonomy and amount of time available for nonprofessional activities, and only 24% were satisfied with the hours spent on administrative activities [40]. A survey of Massachusetts primary care physicians found that 33% were dissatisfied with their practice situation in 1999 compared with 20% in 1996 [41]. Twenty-two percent of primary care physicians in small offices—which provide about half of primary care in the United States—were dissatisfied with the practice of medicine in 2000–2001. Twenty-two percent of all primary care physicians did not feel they could provide high-quality care to all their patients [42].

Morrison and Smith have termed the current predicament in health care *hamster health care*:

> Across the globe doctors are miserable because they feel like hamsters on a treadmill. They must run faster just to stand still... But systems that depend on everybody running faster are not sustainable. The answer must be to redesign health care...The result of the wheel going faster is not only a reduction in the quality of care but also a reduction in professional satisfaction and an increase in burnout among doctors [43].

Declining Interest in Adult Primary Care Careers

In 1992, 1398 graduates of U.S. allopathic medical schools entered family medicine residency programs. This number rose to 2340 in 1997, when it peaked and started downward. In 2005, only 1132 graduates of U.S. medical schools entered family medicine residencies. The total number of first-year residency positions in family medicine had declined from 2905 in 1997 to 2292 in 2005, with international medical graduates filling 48% of the slots. The percent of all U.S. medical graduates choosing family medicine had dropped from 14% in 2000 to 8% in 2005 [44].

Analyzing the choice of a primary care internal medicine career is more difficult since some medical graduates who enter internal medicine residencies end up in primary care while others move on to medical subspecialties. The total number of graduates of U.S. medical schools choosing all internal medicine residencies had fallen only slightly from 2798 in 2001 to 2659 in 2005 [45]. However, whereas half of internal medicine residents previously selected primary care medicine, currently 75–80% of these residents opt for subspecialties (e.g., cardiology, pulmonary medicine, endocrinology, nephrology) [46]. A few internal medicine residency slots are dedicated for primary care, but the number of medical graduates entering these residencies declined from 369 in 2001 to 280 in 2005. U.S. medical schools contributed 170 of the 280 first-year 2005 primary care internal medicine residents [45].

Several factors explain medical graduates' decreasing interest in primary care. One is the uncontrollable lifestyle required by primary care, with long work hours and frequent night call [47]. Another is the low income of primary care physicians, compared with that of many specialists, a factor compounded by the high level of medical school indebtedness. Yet another factor is a medical education environment that promotes specialization [48]. Perhaps the single greatest challenge to attracting medical students to primary care careers is their awareness that many primary care clinicians are trapped in outmoded practice models, struggling to meet seemingly unmanageable clinical expectations in practice settings poorly designed to accomplish the essential and growing tasks of primary care. Forty-six percent of primary care physicians work in offices of four physicians or less [49]. Whereas larger primary care sites often employ nurses, health educators, and other health professionals, the small practices are usually staffed by a small number of receptionists and medical assistants who have not received professional training. The potential for innovation in primary care practice appears far more limited in the small practice milieu.

Patients' Difficulty Obtaining Appointments

A 1999 survey of insured adults younger than 65 years found that 27% of people with health problems had difficulty gaining timely access to a clinician [50]. From 1997 to 2001, the percentage of people reporting an inability to obtain a timely appointment rose from 23% to 33% [51]. In 2001, 43% of adults reporting an urgent condition were sometimes unable to receive care as soon as they wanted [52].

Inconsistent Quality of Care

Half of the patients hospitalized with congestive heart failure are read-mitted within 90 days [53]. Sixty-three percent of people with diabetes have Hb A1c levels greater than 7% [54]. Sixty-six percent of people with hypertension have poorly controlled blood pressures [55]. Only half of tobacco users are counseled about smoking cessation by their physician [56]. Similarly distressing statistics can be found for patients with chronic atrial fibrillation, asthma, and depression [57]. In a large national evaluation of physician performance on 439 quality indicators for 30 medical conditions, patients received only 55% of recommended care [58].

Primary care physicians are not solely responsible for these types of deficiencies, and in fact, appear to perform as well as do specialists caring for patients with common chronic illnesses [24]. However, most chronic care visits take place in primary care offices: 85% for chronic obstructive pulmonary disease, 82% for hypertension, 68% for diabetes, 58% for stroke, 57% for coronary artery disease, and 56% for asthma [59].

The rates of providing clinical preventive services recommended by national guidelines are also not up to par. In a study of 4049 patient visits provided by 138 family physicians, patients were up-to-date on 55% of routine screening tests, 24% of immunizations, and 9% of health-habit counseling services [60].

Increased Responsibilities with Short Visit Times

Over the past two decades, primary care physicians have faced a huge increase in clinical responsibilities [1]. Four new vaccines (*Haemophilus influenzae*, hepatitis B, varicella, and pneumococcus) have been introduced into the routine childhood immunization series. Adult immunizations—hepatitis, pneumococcus, and influenza—came of age during the same era. A few decades ago, cancer screening was limited to Papanicolaou tests. Currently, screening for breast, colon, and prostate cancer consti-tutes routine primary care practice, with considerable patient education required to discuss the risks and benefits of prostate-specific antigen testing, the appropriate age range for mammography, and the appropriate colon cancer screening technique—stool hemoccult, sigmoidoscopy, or colonoscopy.

Management of many illnesses has become far more complicated. Care for patients with diabetes illustrates growing demands in chronic illness care. An aging, more sedentary, more obese U.S. population has developed a greater prevalence of type 2 diabetes mellitus. More aggressive screening combined with less restrictive criteria for diagnosing diabetes has resulted in earlier detection. Until recently, lack of convenient methods for home blood glucose level monitoring and lack of evidence about the effectiveness of tight glycemic control made loose control of blood glucose an acceptable practice via rudimentary monitoring of urine glucose and ketone levels. Before the 1980s, routine Hb A1c testing did not exist, much less guidelines for periodic testing, annual eye examinations, blood pressure control, and lipid management. In the premanaged-care era, a nonketotic patient with hyperglycemia could spend several days in the hospital for treatment and diabetic education, in contrast with the current expectation for intensive treatment and teaching in ambulatory and home settings. An aging population with a greater prevalence of chronic disease means that physicians often must manage multiple illnesses in the same patient.

The scope of primary care practice has also expanded in the face of growing medicalization of social problems. Depression and other forms of mental illness are increasingly recognized as benefiting from appropriate diagnosis and medical treatment. School problems that once earned only detentions now generate queries to the primary care physician about attention-deficit disorder. Primary care physicians are expected to screen patients for substance abuse, domestic violence, and HIV (human immunodeficiency virus) risk behaviors. Even snoring is no longer considered a benign, annoying behavior, but must be evaluated as a possible symptom of sleep apnea, with its attendant complications of arterial and pulmonary hypertension.

Family physicians manage an average of 3.05 clinical problems per encounter; the average is 3.88 for patients older than 65 years and 4.60 for patients with diabetes [61].

Faced with these demands, primary care physicians sense that patient care visits are becoming more rushed. In a nationwide survey of 12,000 physicians, 42% of primary care physicians reported not having adequate time to spend with their patients in 2000–2001, up from 33% in 1996–1997 [42].

Shorter visit times have been associated with reduced quality of care [62, 63], and lower patient and physician satisfaction [64, 65].

Despite the perception of many primary care physicians that visit times are becoming shorter, the real problem may be less a matter of shorter visits than a growing mismatch between clinical demands and the time allotted for the traditional office visit. Between 1989 and 1998, average face-to-face visit times in the United States actually increased by more than 1 minute [66]. However, primary care physicians face far more demands, than in the past, on what they are being called on to deliver in the office visit. They are being profiled, and in part being paid, based on the quality of their practice. Yet the time required to furnish a typical panel of 2500 patients with all recommended preventive care would take 7.4 hours per working day [67]. Additionally, it would take an estimated 10.6 hours per day to adequately manage a similar panel's chronic conditions [68]. Presumably, primary care physicians could spend the remaining 6 hours of each 24-hour day attending to patients' actual symptoms! For primary care physicians, living up to expectations has become close to impossible.

Inadequate Reimbursement

Because of inadequate reimbursement, many primary care physicians are under pressure to care for excessively large patient panels, which leads to reduced timely access to appointments and short visit times. Median primary care income was $157,000 in 2003 compared with $296,000 for specialists. In some cities, primary care physicians face long and intense work days while their income has remained around $100,000 for several years. Between 1999 and 2003, compensation for primary care physicians went up 9% with their productivity rising 25%, indicating that they are working harder for the same inflation-adjusted income. Specialist compensation during those years rose 21% [69].

CAN PRIMARY CARE FULFILL ITS VISION?

Primary care's vision is embodied in the four pillars holding up the primary care home: first-contact care, continuity over time, comprehensiveness, and coordination. Through patients' eyes, the vision promises "If I get sick I can see my primary care physician soon; I have been seeing her for many years; she takes care of most of my medical problems; and if I need other doctors, hospitals, pharmacies, or other care outside her office, she organizes it."

Is primary care fulfilling this vision?

- First-contact care: In 2001, 33% of people surveyed were unable to obtain a timely appointment [51].
- Continuity over time: Only about 50% of patients in several studies report consistently seeing the same physician [70].
- Comprehensiveness: If primary care physicians with panels of 2500 patients need to spend 7.4 hours per day providing evidence-based preventive services [67] and 10.6 hours per day managing chronic illnesses [68], comprehensiveness (even with a considerably smaller panel) is beyond the reach of primary care physicians.
- Coordination: A number of studies have found that primary care physicians often provide insufficient information in specialty referrals [4].

Primary care in the United States is currently not able to fulfill its vision.

PUTTING THE PRIMARY CARE HOUSE IN ORDER

Dr. Rebecca Rushmore takes 3 months away from practice. It was hard to get away, and the physician temporarily taking her place was not ideal. But it had to be done. Dr. Rushmore takes yoga classes, learns relaxation techniques, and visits primary care practices that are trying new ideas. The Future of Family Medicine report helps her refocus her thinking, as do people at the Institute for Healthcare Improvement and the microsystems group at Dartmouth Medical School. When she returns to her medical practice, she is determined to make it work for the patients, the staff, and herself. She knows it won't be easy.

Primary care can make its vision come true. To do so, primary care physicians must step off the hamster treadmill and join together with their colleagues and office staff to launch practice innovations.

Primary care physicians need a new environment in which to function, a climate less permeated with stress and overwork. This new environment must be intertwined with systems of care that improve access and quality while relieving physicians' workload. These changes must take place without major increases in total health care costs, requiring an extensive redistribution of health care dollars from specialty and hospital care to a redesigned primary care home.

What are the alternatives to refurbishing the primary care home? What if entry of new medical graduates into primary care specialties continues its downward trajectory leading to a dearth of generalist physicians? One alternative is a system of care that relies almost exclusively on specialist physicians. Fifty percent of chronic disease patients with more than one chronic condition would need to participate in separate, disease-specific programs rather than rely on an integrated primary care approach. Patients would be responsible for initiating and arranging preventive care services through direct-access mammography and colonoscopy centers, pharmacy-based influenza immunization sites, and other preventive care venues. Comprehensiveness, coordination, and care of the whole person would not be dominant values of this system.

Another scenario entails physicians vacating the primary care home to nonphysician clinicians. An exhausted, underpaid cadre of primary care physicians would retire and be replaced by nurse practitioners and other nonphysician clinicians, whose numbers are increasing. A vestigial primary care physician workforce would attempt to bridge the services provided by nonphysician primary practitioners and specialist physicians. The new generation of nonphysician clinicians would struggle with the same irrationalities and dysfunctional systems that drove physicians from primary care practice.

Neither of these scenarios is satisfactory. All health systems need a sturdy primary care home. Although physicians will not play as dominant a primary care role as they once did, future care models configured around multidisciplinary teams will require physicians' strong and continued presence.

The need for internal redesign does not mean that external factors should be belittled or overlooked. The United States needs to drastically reduce the income disparities between generalist and specialist physicians, link small physician practices into loosely or tightly organized systems, and avoid needless administrative complexity. Yet even if external storms ceased to buffet the primary care home, primary care needs to get its internal house in order.

Many primary care practices in the United States and around the world are reinventing themselves, instituting the innovations described in this book. In the words of Donald Berwick, "We are carrying the 19th-century clinical office into the 21st-century world. It's time to retire it" [71].

REFERENCES

1. Grumbach K, Bodenheimer T: A primary care home for Americans: putting the house in order. JAMA. 2002;288:889–893.
2. Institute of Medicine: *Primary Care: America's Health in a New Era.* Washington, DC, National Academy Press; 1996.
3. Grumbach K, Selby JV, Damberg C, et al: Resolving the gatekeeper conundrum. JAMA. 1999;282:261–266.
4. Starfield B: *Primary Care: Balancing Health Needs, Services and Technology.* New York, Oxford University Press; 1998.
5. Bodenheimer T, Lo B, Casalino L: Primary care physicians should be coordinators, not gatekeepers. JAMA. 1999;281:2045–2049.
6. US General Accounting Office: *Physician Workforce.* GAO-04-124. Washington, DC, October 2003.
7. *Physician Assistant and Nurse Practitioner Workforce Trends.* Washington, DC, The Robert Graham Center, October 2005. (*www.graham-center.org*)
8. Graham R, Roberts RG, Ostergaard DJ, et al: Family practice in the United States. JAMA. 2002;288:1097–1101.
9. Parchman ML, Pugh JA, Noel PH, et al: Continuity of care, self-management behaviors, and glucose control in patients with type 2 diabetes. Med Care. 2002;40:137–144.
10. Shea S, Misra D, Ehrlich MH, et al: Predisposing factors for severe, uncontrolled hypertension in an inner-city minority population. N Engl J Med. 1992;327:776–781.
11. Saultz JW, Lochner J: Interpersonal continuity of care and care outcomes: a critical review. Ann Fam Med. 2005;3:159–166.
12. Bindman AB, Grumbach K, Osmond D, et al: Primary care and receipt of preventive services. J Gen Intern Med. 1996;11:269–276.
13. Safran DG, Taira DA, Rogers WH, et al: Linking primary care performance to outcomes of care. J Fam Pract. 1998;47:213–220.
14. Stewart AL, Grumbach K, Osmond DH, et al: Primary care and patient perceptions of access to care. J Fam Pract. 1997;44:177–185.
15. Rosenblatt RA, Hart LG, Baldwin LM, et al: The generalist role of specialty physicians: is there a hidden system of primary care? JAMA. 1998;279:1364–1370.

16. Macinko J, Starfield B, Shi L: The contribution of primary care systems to health outcomes within Organization for Economic Cooperation and Development (OECD) countries, 1970–1998. Health Serv Res. 2003;38:831–865.
17. Starfield B: Deconstructing primary care. In: Showstack J, Rothman AA, Hassmiller SB, eds: *The Future of Primary Care.* San Francisco, CA, Jossey-Bass; 2004.
18. Ferrer RL, Hambidge SJ, Maly, RC: The essential role of generalists in health care systems. Ann Intern Med. 2005;142:691–699.
19. Fryer GE, Consoli R, Miyoshi TJ, et al: Specialist physicians providing primary care services in Colorado. J Am Board Fam Pract. 2004;17:81–90.
20. Koopman RJ, May KM: Specialist management and coordination of "out-of-domain care." Fam Med. 2004;36:46–50.
21. Weiss LJ, Blustein J: Faithful patients: The effect of long-term physician-patient relationships on the costs and use of health care by older Americans. Am J Public Health. 1996;86:1742–1747.
22. De Maeseneer JM, De Prins L, Gosset H, et al: Provider continuity in family medicine: does it make a difference for total health care costs? Ann Fam Med. 2003;1:144–148.
23. Greenfield S, Nelson EC, Zubkoff M, et al: Variations in resource utilization among medical specialties and systems of care. JAMA. 1992;267: 1624–1630.
24. Greenfield S, Rogers W, Mangotich M, et al: Outcomes of patients with hypertension and non–insulin-dependent diabetes mellitus treated by different systems and specialties: results from the medical outcomes study. JAMA. 1995;274:1436–1444.
25. Carey TS, Garrett J, Jackman A, et al: The outcomes and costs of care for acute low back pain among patients seen by primary care practitioners, chiropractors, and orthopedic surgeons. N Engl J Med. 1995;333:913–917.
26. Harrold LR, Field TS, Gurwitz JH, et al: Knowledge, patterns of care, and outcomes of care for generalists and specialists. J Gen Intern Med. 1999;14: 499–511.
27. Parchman ML, Culler S: Primary care physicians and avoidable hospitalizations. J Fam Pract. 1994;39:123–128.
28. Welch WP, Miller ME, Welch HG, et al: Geographic variation in expenditures for physicians' services in the United States. N Engl J Med. 1993;328: 621–627.
29. Fisher ES, Wennberg DE, Stukel TA, et al: The implications of regional variations in Medicare spending. Ann Intern Med. 2003;138:273–287, 288–298.
30. Fisher ES: Medical care—is more always better? N Engl J Med. 2003;349: 1665–1667.
31. Baicker K, Chandra A: Medicare spending, the physician workforce, and beneficiaries' quality of care. Health Aff Web Exclusive. 2004;W4-184–197.

32. Safran DG: Defining the future of primary care: what can we learn from patients? Ann Intern Med. 2003;138:248–255.
33. Robinson JC: The end of managed care. JAMA. 2001;285:2622–2628.
34. St. Peter RF, Reed MC, Kemper P. et al: Changes in the scope of care provided by primary care physicians. N Engl J Med. 1999;341:1980–1985.
35. Moore GT: Primary care in crisis, in Showstack J, Rothman AA, Hassmiller SB, eds: *The Future of Primary Care.* San Francisco, CA, Jossey-Bass, 2004.
36. Mullan F: Primary care: an endangered species? *The National AHEC Bulletin.* 2000;17(2):1, 6–9.
37. *The Future of General Practice.* London, Royal College of General Practitioners. 2004.
38. Landon BE, Reschovsky J, Blumenthal D: Changes in career satisfaction among primary care and specialist physicians, 1997–2001. JAMA. 2003;289:442–449.
39. Grumbach K, Dower C, Mutha S, et al: *California Physicians 2002: Practice and Perceptions.* San Francisco, CA, UCSF Center for the Health Professions, 2002.
40. Kaiser Family Foundation: National Survey of Physicians, 2002.
41. Landon BE, Aseltine R, Shaul FA, et al: Evolving dissatisfaction among primary care physicians. Am J Manag Care . 2002;8:890–901.
42. Center for Studying Health System Change Physician Survey: (*http://CTSonline.s-3.com/psurvey.asp*)
43. Morrison I, Smith R: Hamster health care: time to stop running faster and redesign health care. BMJ. 2000;321:1541–1542.
44. Pugno PA, Schmittling GT, Fetter GT, et al: Results of the 2005 national resident matching program: family medicine. Fam Med. 2005;37:555–564.
45. Data from the National Resident Matching Program, 2005. (*www.nrmp.org*)
46. Gesensway D: Internal medicine programs maintain a steady draw in this year's match. ACP Observer. 2005. (*www.acponline.org*)
47. Dorsey ER, Jarjoura D, Rutecki GW, et al: Influence of controllable lifestyle on recent trends in specialty choice by U.S. medical students. JAMA. 2003;290:1173–1178.
48. Whitcomb ME, Cohen JJ: The future of primary care medicine. N Engl J Med. 2004;351:710–712.
49. Kane CK: The practice arrangements of patient care physicians, 1999. Chicago: American Medical Association Center for Health Policy Research, 2001; and personal communication, Carol Kane, AMA Center for Health Policy Research.
50. National Survey of Consumer Experiences With Health Plans. Menlo Park, CA, Kaiser Family Foundation; June 2000.
51. Strunk BC, Cunningham PJ: *Treading water: Americans' access to needed medical care*, 1997–2001. Washington, DC, Center for Studying Health System Change. 2002.

52. Greenblatt J: Access to Urgent Medical Care, 2001. Rockville, Md: Agency for Healthcare Research and Quality, 2002. Statistical brief No. 08.
53. Ni H, Nauman DJ, Hershberger RE: Managed care and outcomes of hospitalization among elderly patients with congestive heart failure. Arch Intern Med. 1998;158:1231–1236.
54. Saydah SH, Fradkin J, Cowie CC: Poor control of risk factors for vascular disease among adults with previously diagnosed diabetes. JAMA. 2004;291: 335–342.
55. Chobanian AV, Bakris GL, Black HR, et al: The seventh report of the Joint National Committee on Prevention, Detection, Evaluation, and Treatment of High Blood Pressure. JAMA. 2003;289:2560–2572.
56. Perez-Stable EJ, Fuentes-Afflick E: Role of clinicians in cigarette smoking prevention. West J Med. 1998;169:23–29.
57. Bodenheimer T: Interventions to improve chronic illness care: evaluating their effectiveness. Dis Manag . 2003;6:63–71.
58. McGlynn EQ, Asch SM, Adams J, et al: The quality of health care delivered to adults in the United States. N Engl J Med. 2003;348:2635–2645.
59. Green LA: Is primary care worthy of physicians? An ecological perspective. In: Showstack J, Rothman AA, Hassmiller SB, eds: *The Future of Primary Care.* San Francisco, Jossey-Bass; 2004.
60. Stange KC, Flocke SA, Goodwin MA, et al: Direct observation of rates of preventive service delivery in community family practice. Prev Med. 2000;31:167–176.
61. Beasley JW, Hankey TH, Erickson R, et al: How many problems do family physicians manage at each encounter? Ann Fam Med. 2004;2:405–410.
62. Zyzanski SJ, Stange KC, Langa D, et al: Trade-offs in high-volume primary care practice. J Fam Pract. 1998;46:397–402.
63. Dugdale DC, Epstein R, Pantilat SZ: Time and the physician-patient relationship. J Gen Intern Med. 1999;14(Suppl 1):S34–S40.
64. Mechanic D: Physician discontent. JAMA. 2003;290:941–946.
65. Wetterneck TB, Linzer M, McMurray JE, et al: Worklife and satisfaction of general internists. Arch Intern Med. 2002;162:649–656.
66. Mechanic D, McAlpine DD, Rosenthal M: Are patients' office visits with physicians getting shorter? N Engl J Med. 2001;344:198–204.
67. Yarnall KS, Pollak KI, Ostbye T, et al: Primary care: is there enough time for prevention? Am J Public Health. 2003;93:635–41.
68. Ostbye T, Yarnall KS, Krause KM, et al: Is there time for management of patients with chronic diseases in primary care? Ann Fam Med. 2005;3: 209–14.
69. American Medical News, Sept 20, 2004.
70. Nutting PA, Goodwin MA, Flocke SA, et al: Continuity of primary care: to whom does it matter and when? Ann Fam Med. 2003;1:149–155.
71. Lippman H: Practice in the twenty-first century. *Hippocrates.* 2000:38–43.

CHAPTER TWO

A New Practice Model for Primary Care

How should the primary care practice of the twenty-first century look? Over the past few years, a number of organizations have helped to paint a picture of the future—a New Practice Model for primary care. While it is called the *New Practice Model*, this vision remains anchored on the four traditional pillars of primary care practice: first-contact care, continuity of care over time, comprehensive care, and coordination of care. These foundations of primary care remain as relevant today as when first assembled almost 50 years ago. The New Practice Model proposes new ways to operationalize these principles and makes important additions to traditional primary care.

A key contributor to the New Practice Model was the 2001 Institute of Medicine report, *Crossing the Quality Chasm: A New Health System for the 21st Century*. The *Chasm* report proposed six goals for improvement: that health care be safe, effective, patient-centered, timely, efficient, and equitable. The report suggested macrosystem reforms (e.g., aligning payment of providers with quality improvement) and microsystem improvements (e.g., computerized information technology, health care teams, and advanced access scheduling), but stopped short of prescribing a concrete blueprint for the future.

Seven national family medicine organizations, staffed by the American Academy of Family Physicians, launched the Future of Family Medicine project in 2002 resulting in a similar set of principles for the New

Practice Model. Primary care practices would serve as the personal medical home for every person; practices would adopt a patient-centered team approach, eliminate barriers to access, implement advanced information systems including an electronic health record, focus on quality and outcomes, and enhance practice finance [1]. The Society of General Internal Medicine has endorsed a similar New Practice Model [2].

While the Institute for Healthcare Improvement (IHI) has concentrated on making practical improvements in practices, it has also provided a vision of the future. IHI promotes advanced access, use of Chronic Care Model components to improve quality, patient self-management support, and reduced waste to improve efficiency [3]. A central feature of IHI's visionary leader Donald Berwick is an uncompromising focus on the patient as the central figure in health care [4].

Many primary care practices in the United States and around the world are implementing components of the New Practice Model, particularly in integrated delivery systems, community health centers, some academic medical centers, and publicly organized health systems in other nations. A listing of some innovative primary care practices is provided in Appendix A. Small primary care practices, which care for close to half of primary care patients in the United States, have been less able to muster the time and resources for innovation. In view of the diversity of the settings and innovations currently under way in primary care, the New Practice Model might be more aptly referred to as New Practice Models. Almost certainly, the New Practice Model will not consist of a one-size-fits-all, single-best model, but rather a variety of new models that adapt to their local contexts.

New Practice Models are largely in experimental stages of development. In subsequent chapters, we review some early evidence on the effectiveness of New Practice Model components. In this chapter, we illustrate how one version of a twenty-first century primary care practice might look. Rather than projecting a utopian vision of the New Practice Model, the chapter highlights some of the trade-offs and challenges associated with such a transformation.

BUILDING THE NEW PRACTICE MODEL

Physical Space and Patient Flow

Maria Esperanza was tired. Her workday had started at 6:00 A.M. and she did not look forward to her 3:30 P.M. appointment with Dr. Carolyn

Newhouse. Ms. Esperanza hadn't been to the office for 2 years, but she recalled the long waits in the crowded waiting room filled with coughing patients and crying children. Entering the office door, she couldn't believe her eyes. There was no waiting room.

"Welcome to our redesigned practice," said the receptionist. "Please come into this room so that you can enter your current problems into the touchscreen computer. If you are not comfortable with computers, a medical assistant will help you. Then, if you have to wait, you can go into the patient education room. Videos and interactive programs are available."

Patients coming to primary care should not wait. All the time spent in the practice should be fruitful, using the opportunity for patient education. Some practices have held group educational meetings for patients waiting to see clinicians.

The realities of primary care reimbursement, however, are a major obstacle to this kind of redesign. Space is often in short supply. Inadequate primary care reimbursement makes architectural remodeling and computerization a financial hardship.

The receptionist gave Ms. Esperanza a cycle time form. "We'll write down the exact time you walked in; please enter the time you are seen by the clinician, the time you leave the clinician, and the time you exit the office. Leave the form with us. Our goal is 1 hour from door-in to door-out. You can see from this run chart how our cycle time has been improving."

Many practices have reduced their cycle time and techniques have been developed to implement this improvement (see Appendix G).

Information Technology

Dr. Newhouse and Ms. Esperanza are not the only parties in the room when their clinical visit begins. The computer housing the electronic health record is an active third participant in the encounter. The clinician, patient, and computer sit in a triangular relationship so that the two people can see each other and the computer screen. The history Ms. Esperanza entered into the touch screen is brought up onto the computer screen, and she reviews it with Dr. Newhouse. When the physical exam is complete, Dr. Newhouse enters the findings into the health record allowing Ms. Esperanza to ask questions about what was observed. The two participate in a shared decision-making process about which lab tests and x-rays to perform, based on recommended guidelines, and also about what behavior changes or medications Ms. Esperanza will consider to help improve her health. By the time the encounter is over, all relevant information has been entered into the health record with the patient's review.

The New Model Practice is virtually paperless. Receptionists take down phone messages on computer and route them by e-mail. Medical records are electronic, interfacing with labs, x-ray departments, hospitals, specialists, and pharmacies. Patients are given the choice to access the practice through e-mail or the Internet. Using a clinical triage software program, receptionists can determine if patients need lab work or x-rays prior to a visit, whether their problem can be handled by phone, or how urgently they need to see a clinician. Patient education materials are easily printable from computers in multiple languages. Clinical practice guidelines and algorithms to assist in shared decision-making are swiftly accessible electronically during the clinician visit.

While the advantages of a paperless office are numerous, a number of obstacles must first be confronted as discussed in Chapter 8. Costs are considerable. Creating a digital practice requires a total workflow overhaul of the processes described in Chapter 10. Clinicians often find that entering data into the electronic health record takes longer than writing in a paper chart. Some work that was formerly done by nonclinician staff may become the responsibility of clinicians, which can make the hamster wheel go even faster—the opposite of what was intended. With thought and ingenuity these barriers can be overcome.

Primary care teams

Ms. Esperanza is invited to a meeting at Dr. Newhouse's practice. She arrives to find seven other patients, three practice clinicians, and a facilitator. The topic of discussion is primary care teams. First, the patients are asked to say what they need from the practice. The concerns are similar: "I want to see my doctor every time I come." "It takes too long to get an appointment." "My visits with the doctor are too short."

Next, the two physicians are asked to say what they need. "I'm working from 7:00 A.M. to 8:00 P.M. and I never have time for my family." "I can't do everything the patients need in the 15-minute visit." "A lot of what I do is routine and could be done by someone else; then I could spend more time with complicated patients." The nurse practitioner, while working fewer hours, echoed the same concerns.

The patients are then invited to respond. The feeling is unanimous— what we need is very different from, and even to a degree antagonistic to, what the clinicians need. There need to be some compromises.

Dr. Newhouse then summarizes a proposal that the practice is considering—to reorganize care into teams. The practice would be divided into two teams, each with two part-time physicians, one nurse practitioner, three medical assistants, and one receptionist. Each patient would have a personal clinician—either a physician or nurse practitioner—and would be a patient of one team. The practice would attempt to offer continuity of care with the personal clinician but would not guarantee it. The practice would promise that patients would always be seen by someone on their team. Phone calls would be routed to the receptionist of the patient's team.

At that point, a lively discussion ensued, with patients voicing concern that they might not like other team members, and that they would still have long waits for appointments and short visit times. They took a straw vote and accepted the team concept. So far, the process was working.

Then Dr. Newhouse opened Pandora's box. "Many patients are healthy, or have high blood pressure, diabetes, high cholesterol, and other chronic conditions or risk factors that are stable. With all the things that clinicians need to think about, it makes sense for other members of the staff to be responsible for routine preventive and chronic care. We are therefore proposing that the medical assistants take over these routine tasks. A healthy person would make an appointment with the medical assistant once a year, would have evidence-based studies and immunizations ordered, and would come back to see the nurse practitioner for results and health concerns. The same process would take place for patients with stable chronic conditions, except that the visits would be more frequent, depending on practice guidelines. For each team, one medical assistant each day would be freed of her usual duties to provide time for routine chronic and preventive care."

All hell broke loose. "We've heard about diabetes and cholesterol and how they are spreading among our youth. We need doctors to stop this epidemic." "My daughter is a medical assistant. She went to school for 6 months. She knows nothing. I bet half the blood pressures she takes are wrong."

After a heated discussion, the facilitator made a proposal. The practice would do some Plan-Do-Study-Act (PDSA) practice improvement cycles, testing out the idea on a small scale—one medical assistant, one physician, and ten patients with diabetes. One of the nurse practitioners would provide the medical assistant with 2 weeks of training and the physician would prepare protocols—standing orders—for routine diabetes care. The nurse practitioner would observe the medical assistant's visits and mentor her. After 1 month, Dr. Newhouse would meet with the 10 patients to get their feedback.

The atmosphere in the room lightened up. The patients agreed to the experiment provided the idea would be scrapped if patient feedback was negative.

Primary care teams come in many shapes and sizes, depending on available personnel. As discussed in Chapter 9, key components of care teams are measurable goals, delineation of all clinical processes, clear division of labor for each process, training and mentoring, and communication. Physicians are not able to provide all evidence-based acute, chronic, and preventive care in the 15-minute visit. Teams are needed to ensure that all evidence-based care for a patient panel is provided, and the team needs to figure out who will provide which components of the total care package.

In one scenario, the physician's scope of work is reduced by delegating routine chronic and preventive care to other team members. In larger practices, nurses, pharmacists, or health educators could take on these responsibilities. In small offices, medical assistants are the predominant nonclinician team members, though virtual teams with caregivers in hospitals or other practices, interacting electronically or by telephone, are an attractive alternative.

In one version of the New Practice Model, physicians would see only 8–10 (rather than 25–30) patients per day. The physician would spend considerable time training and consulting with other team members. Physician visits, chiefly with complicated patients, would last about 30 minutes, making the encounters meaningful to both patient and physician. Less complex problems would be handled in person, via telephone, or e-mail by nurse practitioners or physician assistants. If available, health educators or nurse educators would perform the time-consuming work of self-management support and behavior change counseling (see Chapter 5). A serious challenge would be to prevent nurse practitioners and physician assistants from becoming the new generation of hamsters.

In this scenario, nurses (in larger practices) or receptionists (in small practices) would become integral members of the clinical team, with intensive training to carry out three functions: (1) to be the triage person within the team, deciding (with help if needed) which patients are seen how urgently by whom; (2) to be the communications person within the team, making sure information is electronically routed to the proper team members (phone messages, calls from outside doctors and nurses, pharmacy calls, lab/x-ray results, and so forth); and (3) if legally permissible, to manage—with oversight—simple medical problems under protocol, for example, colds, uncomplicated urinary tract infections, and certain prescription refills. Personnel providing these functions would need to be relieved of other activities.

Rigorously engineered systems, specifying who does what, would be created for all clinical processes such as prescription refills, referrals, preventive services, management of stable, chronic conditions, sorting incoming e-mails by level of urgency and properly routing them to the appropriate team member, and informing patients of normal and abnormal test results.

The formation of cohesive teams is easier said than done. Personalities may get in the way. Time for training and mentoring is hard to schedule. Turnover among medical assistants and receptionists can lead to hours of training being wasted; on the other hand, integrating practice staff into a clinical team can improve satisfaction and reduce turnover. Licensing and legal issues may restrict the scope of work of nonclinicians.

Patients invariably want physicians to do everything, though good experiences with non-physician care can usually persuade them otherwise. Fee-for-service payment is a barrier of gargantuan proportions, since nonclinician visits are rarely reimbursed. Excessive panel size—too many patients with too many diseases—can sink any effort to form teams because physicians will never be able to reduce their visit load in order to become mentors and trainers.

Patient-Centered Encounters

Ms. Esperanza likes Dr. Newhouse, but has one problem with her. To put it nicely, the doctor moves too fast. Ms. Esperanza bucks up her courage and haltingly confronts Dr. Newhouse. "Doc, I know you only have 15 minutes. I try to be brief in telling you my concerns, but you interrupt me before I get a chance to finish. Then you tell me what tests to get, what changes in my lifestyle you want me to make, and what medications you order me to take. But you go so fast that I can't understand half of what you say. Then you get annoyed at me for not doing what you told me. Also, though I greatly respect your knowledge and concern for me, I don't always want to do the things you advise. I would like to make some of those decisions jointly."

Dr. Newhouse is crushed. She thought she was a good doctor and a caring one. Is Ms. Esperanza one of those hopelessly difficult patients who are never satisfied, or might she be right? Dr. Newhouse leaves the room to collect her thoughts.

These days everyone talks about patient-centered care. But few clinicians understand the specific changes needed to transform the clinician-patient encounter into a patient-centered interaction. Even fewer clinicians, trained in traditional physician-directed care, are able to make the paradigm shift to a clinician-patient partnership. Practical patient-centered concepts are enumerated in Chapters 3, 5, and Appendix L. They include collaborative setting of the visit agenda; *closing the loop* to verify patient understanding of clinician advice; shared decision-making about diagnostic tests and procedures, medications, and surgical interventions; and collaborative goal setting to assist with lifestyle changes.

Even if clinicians are able to make this paradigm shift, they are often unable to implement patient-centered care on a consistent basis because it takes more time. For that reason, a primary care team is a prerequisite to patient-centered care. All team members need to understand patient-centered processes and extra time needs to be made available.

Where will the extra time be found? Any patient who does not need to come to the office should not be there. Donald Berwick estimates that 50–80% of office visits are "neither wanted by the patients nor deeply believed in by the doctor." [5]

When patients who do not want or need to be in the office are in the office, receptionists, medical assistants, and clinicians have more work. Less time is available to offer truly patient-centered care to people who need acute, chronic, or preventive services. The difficulty, of course, is that fee-for-service payment rewards more rather than fewer visits—another reason why the New Practice Model requires payment reform. The New Practice Model cannot be achieved without alternatives to the individual face-to-face visit, along with reform of payment policies to compensate clinicians for alternative encounters.

Alternative Encounters

For far too long, medical care has been stuck on the one-to-one, face-to-face, doctor-patient visit. The New Practice Model expands the types of encounters that patients can choose.

Don Digital, a 29-year-old web designer with ulcerative colitis, comes to Dr. Newhouse with a proposal. He wants to help the practice develop a secure web and e-mail patient portal, and offers to check out the various vendors for the medical practice. He thinks he can find a company who would give the practice a big discount if the practice is willing to discuss the portal with other potential customers.

Many patient needs can be fulfilled without face-to-face visits (see Chapter 7). For years, the telephone has replaced the stethoscope as the most useful tool in medicine; electronic communication is the next powerful tool. Large provider organizations are instituting web portals for patients, and patient-practice e-mail will soon be routine in primary care practice. Patients can use electronic means of communication to make appointments; obtain lab and x-ray results (with explanations of their significance); inform clinicians of home-monitored levels of blood pressures, blood sugars, and weights; arrange prescription refills; and engage in question and answer dialogues with clinicians.

Parallel to the spread of high-tech patient encounters is the even more revolutionary innovation of the low-tech, face-to-face group visit. Group visits allow a vast untapped resource to assist in the care of patients—other patients. When patients in group visits hear the problems of other patients, it places their problems in perspective. Patients with similar illnesses may help each other as much as or more than a physician can help. Patients feel empowered by helping others. In group visits, human interactions are logarithmically multiplied, creating a great potential for healing. A group visit *starter kit* is provided in Appendix I.

An experimental concept, which melds the high-tech and high-interaction innovations, is the web-based group visit.

The barriers to alternative encounters are the usual culprits—money and time. For small primary care practices, the financial investment to put electronic visits in place is considerable. Workflow processes need to be developed such that clinicians have protected time to handle e-communications from patients. Medical assistants or other personnel should be trained to filter and triage e-mails. Group visits require an investment in administrative time and the opportunity for clinicians leading groups to move up the learning curve.

Patient acceptance of alternative modalities is not a problem as long as patients retain choice and are not forced into an uncomfortable type of encounter. However, some patients inappropriately insist on an excessive amount of individual face-to-face time, requiring a major infusion of practice resources. Negotiations with frequent-using patients will be needed to satisfy their needs with fewer practice resources. This difficult issue can be framed as "We are concerned with each patient, but we are also concerned with our entire population of patients. Excessive resources inappropriately concentrated on a few patients leave fewer resources for other patients who may have greater needs."

Population-Based Care

Dr. Newhouse was angry. Her practice received no pay-for-performance bonuses for measures related to the care of patients with diabetes. She was flabbergasted that only 55% of diabetes patients in the practice had received Hb A1c tests in the previous year, and that 40% of those patients had Hb A1c levels greater than 7. She wondered about what might be the Hb A1c levels of patients who had not been tested.

She contacted the American Academy of Family Physicians who referred her to its improvement collaborative on diabetes. The first collaborative learning session featured a presentation on the Chronic Care Model and a workshop on starting a diabetes registry. Dr. Newhouse returned to work, determined to think about the practice's entire panel of patients, rather than focus only on the patients who made appointments.

Patient-centered care may be the most difficult paradigm shift challenging the twenty-first century primary care practice. Another challenging paradigm shift is population-based care. Without a list of who the patients are, what chronic conditions they have, and to what extent those chronic conditions are under optimal control, population-based care is not possible (see Chapter 4). A similar list would identify patients needing preventive-care services. These lists, best created as electronic registries, will become increasingly essential as pay-for-performance takes hold.

Instituting registries as a central activity of primary care requires the usual time and money investment. Ideally, registries are an integral part of the electronic medical record, but not all EMRs (electronic medical records) have this capability. Until a medical office is fully computerized, personnel time is needed to enter data into the registry, and more personnel time is needed to *work* the registry, determining which patients need which services, contacting those patients, and arranging the services to be performed. There is no need for clinicians to be involved in the routine tasks of working the registry.

Planned Care for Patients with Chronic Conditions/Risk Factors

It's happened a hundred times. The 15-minute visit for the woman with diabetes, hypertension, and heart failure. Thirteen minutes spent dealing with acute shoulder pain and insomnia caused by her husband with Alzheimer's disease and two minutes for chronic care management. Dr. Newhouse remembers the Chronic Care Model presentation— planned visits.

The New Practice Model provides lengthy, planned individual or group visits for people with chronic conditions and people needing behavior-change counseling. The problem is: who will lead the planned visits? In larger organizations, nurses, pharmacists, or health educators can be trained as care managers (see Chapter 4). In small practices, nurse practitioners can lead planned visits, but they are often consumed with acute visits. Moreover, if the practice is paid fee-for-service, revenues based on productivity (volume of patients seen) may fall as schedules are partially filled with longer planned visits. Medical assistants, and motivated patients, with proper training, can lead planned visits focusing on behavior-change goal setting (see Chapter 5), but these visits also take considerable personnel time and are rarely reimbursed. While small practices may refer patients for planned visits to the health educator at a nearby hospital, coordination of care between the primary care team and the health educator is more difficult.

Another barrier to planned visits is that many patients show up for care only if they have an acute or poorly controlled chronic problem; they will not make an extra visit for planned care. Attracting patients (especially those less motivated to become good self-managers) to attend planned visits is a problem that few practices have solved.

Patient-Chosen Access

The New Practice Model aims to offer patients appointments when they want or need them (see Chapter 6). Meeting this goal requires that the capacity for providing appointments is equal to the demand for appointments. Usually, practices can sustain patient-chosen access only by reducing the demand for visits through telephone, e-mail, and web encounters. Group visits can increase visit capacity—15 patients in a 2-hour group visit versus 8 patients with 15-minute appointments for 2 hours. A big administrative challenge is balancing patient-chosen access with physicians who devote most of their time to fewer, longer visits with complex patients; the majority of appointment slots will be with nonphysician clinicians, care managers who offer planned visits, and through phone, electronic, or group encounters.

Partnering with Community Organizations

Primary care cannot do it all. Many communities have resources that supplement what primary care can offer, relieving pressure on primary care practices. Exercise programs, senior centers, weight reduction programs, hospital-based patient education, church groups, disease-specific support groups, and other community-based resources can be referral destinations for patients. Many practices are unfamiliar with the range of available resources; cataloguing this information is a time investment that can eventually pay off.

Encouraging Patients to Help

Patients comprise the largest pool of underutilized resources in the health care system. Patients are viewed only as consumers—using up resources. Yet if health care organizations invest in patients through self-management support and training, patients can contribute by healing themselves and helping to heal others. People who are good self-managers utilize the health care system far less than those who consume health care passively [6]; they assist primary care practices by reducing workloads. The Stanford Patient Education Research Center has trained hundreds of patients to lead chronic illness self-management groups, thereby becoming care-givers in addition to care receivers [7]. Patients who have successfully controlled their weight could organize cooking classes for people who need to lose weight. They can lead exercise classes or support groups. Group visits have shown that patients enjoy helping others.

Touching the Patient

The healing power of the laying on of hands has always had great sway. Recently, the concept has surfaced that touching patients has great value, even when the touch is not literally physical contact. A touch is any interaction between a patient and a caregiver (who might be another patient). A face-to-face visit, an e-mail communication, telephone call—all are touches. Strong evidence demonstrates that regular and sustained follow-up is essential for improving ongoing healthy behavior change, medication adherence, and clinical outcomes (see Chapter 5). Maximizing the frequency of follow-up or touches should be an integral part of the New

Practice Model for patients with chronic conditions. For patients who are healthy, staying away—except for periodic preventive services—is good medicine. For the growing numbers of patients with chronic conditions, waiting for them to contact the primary care practice is no longer adequate. The practice needs to touch those patients on a regular basis.

Physicians cannot single-handedly perform all the primary care touches necessary for their panel of patients. Different members of the team must have their hands in the mix when it comes to patient touches, whether it be planned visits, follow-up emails and phone calls, or administering immunizations. One of the major questions facing the New Practice Model is whether the patient-physician relationship will suffer as the physician delegates more touches to other members of the primary care team. Do face-to-face visits, for routine preventive and chronic care services, help build trust and familiarity between patients and physicians that pays off when a patient experiences a major illness, or when a patient needs to confide in the physician about sensitive issues such as mental illness or substance use? Can e-mail and telephone touches build therapeutic alliances, or is the regular laying on of hands necessary for healing relationships? The answers to these questions will be critical to understanding the viability of the New Practice Model.

IS THE NEW PRACTICE MODEL FEASIBLE?

A vision of the future can be enticing. A model—blueprint of a new way—stimulates the intellect. A paradigm shift can create an epiphany.

But primary care faces serious challenges. Visions, models, and epiphanies don't pay the mortgage. *Feasible* is the pertinent adjective.

To implement any component of the New Practice Model, several questions should be asked:

1. Is it financially viable? Does it increase revenues and/or reduce expenses?

2. Does it increase patient satisfaction, clinician satisfaction, staff satisfaction?

3. Is information technology available to make the improvement without a crippling financial investment?

4. Does it improve quality without placing unreasonable new demands on clinician workload?

5. Does it improve access without placing unreasonable new demands on clinician workload?

6. Is there evidence from other organizations or research studies that the improvement can be successful? Who else has done this and what happened?

7. How difficult is it to make the improvement?

8. What tools are available (experiences of other practices, materials, protocols) to assist in making the improvement?

9. What resources are needed to make the improvement? Personnel, management, leadership, IT, money, training time? Are those resources available?

10. Is the improvement compliant with regulations and laws?

11. Is health policy advocacy needed to change the larger health system in order to institute the practice improvement? For example, do reimbursement policies of payers (Medicare, insurers) support or hinder the improvement?

Questions like these are not meant to discourage innovation, but to heighten the chance that innovation will succeed.

The most compelling argument that the New Practice Model is feasible is the success of many primary care practices—in the United States and around the world—in making substantial progress. Any primary care practice ready to begin the journey toward the New Practice Model would best visit one or more of these organizations (see Appendix A).

A saying goes: "How do you eat an elephant?" "One bite at a time." Microsystem analysis (see Chapter 10) provides an approach to a bite-by-bite improvement path, eventually leading toward the New Practice Model. Some tools for practice improvement are provided in Appendices B, C, D, E, G, H, and I.

A worldwide movement is growing to reenergize primary care. This movement has a vision, a set of goals, initial research suggesting that the vision has a basis in evidence, strong leadership, a beginning track record, and the support of some influential organizations. These positive developments provide hope that the storm clouds currently threatening primary care may one day blow over, illuminating primary care with the bright future it deserves.

References

1. Future of Family Medicine Project Leadership Committee: The future of family medicine. Ann Fam Med. 2004;2(Suppl. 1):S3–S32.
2. Society of General Internal Medicine: *The Future of General Internal Medicine*. 2003. (*www.sgim.org/futureofGIMreport.cfm*)
3. (*www.ihi.org*)
4. Berwick DM: Escape Fire. *Designs for the Future of Health Care*. San Francisco, CA, Jossey-Bass, 2004.
5. Wysocki B: Doctor leads a crusade to replace office visits as standard procedure. *Wall Street Journal*,. May 30, 2002, p. 1.
6. Wasson J: *How's Your Health? What You Can Do to Make Your Health and Health Care Better*. FNX Corporation, Lebanon, NH, 2005.
7. (*http://patienteducation.stanford.edu*)

CHAPTER THREE

Patient-Centered Care: Finding the Balance

Patient-centered care is universally supported by health system leaders. Patient centeredness is a basic ingredient of the Institute of Medicine's twenty-first century health system [1]. The Future of Family Medicine project, the Society of General Internal Medicine's report on the future of general internal medicine, and the American College of Physicians' *Prescription for Change* document espouse patient-centered care as a key component of primary care [2–4].

For primary care practices to adopt patient-centered care, however, is a major challenge. This chapter both reviews the elements of patient-centered care and explores the difficulties inherent in its implementation.

Patient-centered care can take place in three interrelated orbits: the inner orbit of the clinician-patient relationship, the surrounding orbit of the medical practice (also known as the *microsystem* as discussed in Chapter 10), and the outermost large health care macrosystem (Figure 3–1). This chapter explores patient-centered care in these three realms.

WHAT IS PATIENT-CENTERED CARE?

The notion of patient-centered care developed to a large degree as a reaction to the problematic features of doctor-centric care and the legacy of overly paternalistic relationships between physicians and their patients.

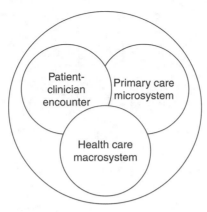

FIGURE 3–1.   Three domains of patient-centered care.

The visit wasn't going well. Dr. Frances Blinder needed to deal with the rise in the cholesterol level and the uncontrolled blood pressure. But Mr. Randall Cross was hell-bent on getting his disability form filled out. "I told him I would do it, but not today," explained Dr. Blinder. "He didn't listen. He was obsessed with that form. He refused to discuss the high blood pressure that was his real problem, and got ready to leave the room. I stayed firm; I sure wasn't going to back down now." Mr. Cross walked out.

On the other hand, the opposite extreme of a *consumerist* relationship between physician and patient, in which the physician provides information and all the decision-making responsibility lies with the patient, also has its drawbacks.

Dr. Buddy Sweet had just returned from a patient empowerment workshop. He was eager to try out the new ideas. Ms. Julia Kay came in, weak and dizzy. Dr. Sweet's associate had called her to come urgently because yesterday's potassium was 2.2. Dr. Sweet was excited. "I'll give her all the options and she can decide." He made a clear list for Ms. Kay: take potassium pills, drink orange juice, or stop the diuretic. Ms. Kay was afraid to stop the diuretic because she didn't like her feet swelling up; she had tried potassium pills before and they upset her stomach. She promised to drink some orange juice. The following day Dr. Sweet received an urgent call from the coroner. Ms. Kay had been picked up by the paramedics for a cardiac arrhythmia but had died en route to the hospital.

The vignettes illustrate that *patient centered* is not a simple concept. It cannot mean that patients decide matters they are ill equipped to decide, or that clinicians abdicate an active role in working with patients to assure delivery of evidence-based care. On the other hand, the patient needs to be involved in setting agendas and clinical decisions.

Patient-centered care, or the lack of it, is a characteristic not only of the clinician-patient encounter, but also of the patient's experience within the primary care microsystem—the local milieu in which patients, providers, support staff, and information converge for the purpose of providing care to meet health needs (see Chapter 10 for more about microsystems).

Lakeisha Jefferson loved her doctor. But the practice staff drove her crazy. She counted 15 minutes on hold for many phone calls. Sometimes after 5 or 10 minutes she would be disconnected. The front office staff never smiled and rarely said hello. The medical assistant never remembered Lakeisha's name and sometimes the wrong chart was pulled for her visit. The billing department got it wrong at least half the time. She couldn't take it any more and reluctantly looked for another doctor.

As Lakeisha Jefferson discovered, a patient-centered encounter with a physician may not be adequate if the clinical microsystem in which the clinician practices is not patient centered.

Clinicians and their microsystems traditionally have held all the cards—the knowledge, the specialty referral form, the request slip for an MRI (magnetic resonance imaging), the prescription pad, and so on. Physicians rarely change their schedules to accommodate the patient's schedule; it is the patient who defers to the doctor's needs. In the microsystem, the practice also tends to hold the cards—providing appointments, allowing telephone access to the clinician, informing the patient of lab and x-ray results, and creating an environment in which the patient feels welcome.

Most patients desire a more empowered relationship with their clinicians and microsystems [5, 6]. For example, research indicates that most patients want to actively participate in medical decisions. Although older and less-educated patients report somewhat less preference for shared decision making, and patients who are critically ill appear more willing to defer to their physician, the majority of patients wish to be involved in treatment decisions [7, 8]. Moreover, there is some evidence that patient outcomes are better when there is more patient-centered care [9]. Patient-centered care has been associated with lower costs for diagnostic testing [10]. Patients also desire that the microsystem be more patient responsive [11, 12].

Some of the lopsidedness in these relationships is necessary and unavoidable; a health system organized entirely around the patient or completely patient-driven would not work. Clinicians do have more knowledge, and their judgment is a vital component of health care. A primary care clinician cannot be accessible 24/7 for his or her patients. Visit lengths and appointment slots are determined not only by patients' preferences, but by clinicians' available time and financial sustainability of the practice. Just as a completely consumerist model for the patient-clinician relationship is not optimal, taken to its extreme the pursuit of a patient-centered microsystem can turn into a counterproductive preoccupation, with superficial elements of customer service at the expense of assuring delivery of evidence-based care.

Patient-centered care seeks a common ground between patient and clinician, and between patients and the health care system. Finding this common ground requires greater patient empowerment, but also an ongoing negotiation to find a balance among the needs and preferences of individual patients, the overall population of patients needing care, and the clinicians and microsystems caring for these patients. Patient-clinician partnership might be a more appropriate term than patient-centered care.

The following section examines specific components of patient-centered care.

PATIENT-CENTERED CARE IN THE PATIENT-CLINICIAN ENCOUNTER

Although there is no universally accepted definition of patient-centered care, there is an agreement that important features include encouraging patients to be more participatory, sharing power and responsibility, supporting patient autonomy and individuality, and attending to the clinician-patient relationship [10, 13]. Practical ways to achieve these patient-centered objectives in the primary care encounter include:

- Agenda setting
- Information exchange
- Shared decision making

Agenda Setting

The vignette about Mr. Cross and Dr. Blinder demonstrates the importance of agenda setting in striving for patient-centered clinical encounters. In actual practice, agenda setting is usually a physician-dominated process. Marvel et al. studied 264 visits to family physicians. Patients making an initial statement of their problem were interrupted by the physician after an average of 23 seconds. In only 28% of the visits were patients able to express their concerns completely. In 25% of the visits, the physician never asked the patient for his or her concerns at all [14]. Another study corroborates this data, finding that patients were interrupted after a mean time of 18 seconds [15].

When clinicians ask patients what they wish to get from the visit, and when clinicians clearly express what they hope to accomplish from the visit, an agenda can be negotiated (see Appendix L). Because of time pressures, each party may need to compromise. However, making the agenda-setting process more explicit does help to level the playing field between the clinician and patient.

Information Exchange

Information exchange is a key part of the primary care encounter and providing information can influence patients' health decisions and behavior. Patients with back pain, who reported that their physicians adequately explained their symptoms, demanded fewer diagnostic tests and were as satisfied as those who received tests [16]. However, research has also revealed important problems in how information is exchanged during visits. As many as 50% of patients leave an office visit not understanding what they were told by the physician [17]. In a study of over 300 medical encounters, physicians devoted an average of 1.3 minutes to giving information, with 88% of the information worded in technical language [18]. In another study, only 37% of patients were adequately informed about medications they were prescribed [19]. Patients not taking their medications as prescribed is most frequently due to miscommunication from physician to patient [20]. In one study, 50% of patients on chronic warfarin therapy had a different idea than their physician about the doses of warfarin they should be taking [21]. Minority patients receive less information about tests, procedures, treatments, and prognosis than White patients [22].

Closing the loop or *teach-back* is a technique to assess patients' understanding of information provided by the clinician (see Chapter 5); clinicians ask patients to restate the information given to see whether the information was understood. In one study, physicians assessed patients' understanding (*closed the loop*) in only 12% of discussions of new information, and when the understanding was assessed, patients had misunderstood 47% of the time. *Closing the loop* was also associated with improved

Hb A1c levels in patients with diabetes [23]. A closing-the-loop discussion example is provided in Appendix L.

Shared Decision Making

Susan Yu was looking for help. For 3 years, the pain in her lower back had limited her activities and interrupted her life. Her friend recommended a primary care group that had a special program for patients with chronic back pain. On the day of the visit, Ms. Yu first met with a physical therapist who was part of the clinic team. The therapist asked many questions about Ms. Yu's back, reviewed the x-ray and MRI scan results, and discussed several options. Then she asked Ms. Yu to view the video Chronic Low Back Pain: Managing Your Pain and Your Life produced by the Foundation for Informed Medical Decision Making and Health Dialog. After the video, the primary care physician joined Ms. Yu and the physical therapist, reviewed the history, performed a brief confirmatory exam, and asked Ms. Yu about her preferences for treatment. The session ended with Ms. Yu rejecting the surgical and steroid injection options and making an action plan involving exercise, yoga, jacuzzi, and acetaminophen. A follow-up meeting was scheduled for 1 month with the physical therapist.

Braddock et al. studied over 1000 audiotaped visits with 59 primary care physicians and 65 surgeons in community practice. In 91% of decisions made in those visits, the patient was not truly informed of the options and consequences related to the decision, i.e., the patient was not engaged in shared decision making [24]. Surgeons did slightly better than primary care physicians. Other studies measuring multidimensional aspects of shared decision making have found somewhat better ratings of shared decision making in practice, although demonstrating considerable room for improvement. Shared decision making also appears to occur less often in visits by minority and low-income patients. One study found that African-American patients cared for by African-American physicians reported greater involvement in medical decisions, more partnership with the physician, and greater trust in the physician than African Americans cared for by White physicians [25].

Several patient-centered interventions can facilitate shared decision making; two of these include preactivation and patient decision aids.

Preactivation: Patient activation refers to patients being active participants in their care (see Chapter 5). Preactivation describes a process of assisting patients to be more assertive in the medical care visit. It can be accomplished by previsit face-to-face discussions, written materials, or computer interactions.

Several randomized trials of preactivation interventions have been performed, including previsit meetings with health educators and interactive training booklets. The interventions attempted to help patients formulate questions in advance of a visit and encouraged them to negotiate decisions with the physician. Most studies found that preactivated patients were more participatory in the visit, had improvements in health-related behaviors, and in some cases had better disease outcomes [26–29]. However, one study uncovered a potential downside to preactivation. In this study, the visits for preactivated patients were characterized by more anxiety and anger, and the patients were less satisfied. It was hypothesized that preactivated patients had higher expectations, which physicians were not able to satisfy in the time available [30, 31].

Patient Decision Aids: Many clinical decisions are *preference sensitive* because the best choice is (1) not scientifically proven and (2) dependent on patients' values and preferences. The proper antibiotic is the best choice for the treatment of bacterial meningitis; it is not preference sensitive. Management of benign prostatic hypertrophy, on the other hand, could involve surgery, medications, or watchful waiting, depending on patient preference. Shared decision making involves practitioners communicating information on the benefits and harms of the different choices available, discussing patients' preferences, and coming to a decision as a clinician-patient partnership.

To assist the shared decision-making process, the Foundation for Informed Medical Decision Making and Health Dialog have developed over 500 patient decision aids using print, audio, video, or web-based media. Health Dialog also offers trained health coaches to discuss treatment options. A systematic review has found that patient decision aids improve patient knowledge, heighten patient activation, and increase patient satisfaction with the decision. Using patient decision aids is associated with a 21–44% reduction in elective surgeries, without adverse effects on health outcomes and with a reduction in health care costs; the surgeries include coronary revascularization, hysterectomy, back surgery, and prostatectomy [32].

The Therapeutic Alliance

Agenda setting, information exchange, and shared decision making are all facets of patient-clinician communication. Although communication behavior is an important piece of patient-centered care, equally important are the less tangible aspects of the patient-clinician relationship: the mutual trust, empathy, and respect that allow collaboration in care and treatment. These are the elements that create what is often referred to as a *therapeutic alliance*. Patients reporting greater trust, increased satisfaction, and more collaborative relationships with clinicians have increased adherence to medication and treatment regimens and better health outcomes [33].

Developing a therapeutic alliance requires more than patient-centered communication techniques. One recent study videotaped patient-physician visits, and then asked the patients and physicians to observe and comment on the videotape. In some instances, the visit looked good in terms of the observable shared decision-making behavior, but *felt bad*, to either the patient or physician, in terms of their more subjective experience of partnership in the visit. Conversely, in some visits, the shared decision-making behavior *looked bad*, but the patient and physician reported a positive sense of partnership. The researchers concluded that patient-centered care requires attention to *both effective communication style and affective relationship dynamics* [34].

PATIENT-CENTERED CARE IN THE PRIMARY CARE MICROSYSTEM

As the vignette about Lakeisha Jefferson earlier in the chapter illustrated, a patient-centered approach is relevant to the entire practice microsystem and not only to the patient-clinician encounter. There are many ways for a primary care practice to become more patient centered: allowing patients to select the day and time of their appointments themselves and ensuring prompt appointments; timely response to telephone calls and e-mails; short waiting times in the office and on the telephone; multiple ways—face-to-face visits, group visits, phone, e-mail or web—to receive their care depending on patient preference and on the problem at hand; the ability to provide care in the patients' preferred languages; continuity of care; and effective relationships with other parts of the health system to facilitate care coordination.

The subsequent chapters in the book discuss in detail many of the strategies for creating a more patient-centered practice.

PATIENT-CENTERED CARE IN THE HEALTH CARE MACROSYSTEM

Dr. Jack Able, the medical director of a large HMO (Health Maintenance Organization)-based physician group, was a whiz at fixing microsystems. He initiated advanced access scheduling in the group's primary care practices, reduced the cycle time in their orthopedics clinic, and put together a program to reduce medical errors in the HMO's hospitals. But when patients were discharged from the hospital, no one called to check on how they were doing. Patients going to a cardiologist were put on medications that the primary care physician didn't know about. Dr. Able left the group's Practice Improvement and Patient Safety Committee crestfallen, after hearing a critical incident report about a recently discharged patient who was unable to return to the lab to get her warfarin dose checked, and almost died of a gastrointestinal bleed from her drug-induced coagulopathy.

Dr. Louise Master wasn't satisfied. She was one of the primary care physicians on Dr. Able's practice improvement teams, and the ratings from the patient satisfaction monitoring surveys were not showing improvement. Dr. Master decided on a new approach. She imagined a patient, whom she called Esther. She wondered what the problems looked like from Esther's vantage point. She organized a focus group of patients, and quickly realized that patients didn't see health care as a hospital here, a primary care clinic there, a cardiology office somewhere else. Esther viewed health care as whatever she needed to get better. She needed someone to come to her house and explain the complicated directions she had received when she left the hospital. She was infirm and needed transportation. She needed to get the same story, and the same pills, from the different doctors she saw. Dr. Master realized that improvements needed to be organized around Esther, not confined to a particular hospital or clinic.

Most efforts to improve health care quality and access, and foster patient-centered care, take place within silos—a particular hospital, a medical group, or the physicians contracting with a particular health plan. From the patient's viewpoint, silos are nothing more than barriers. Hand-offs from one caregiver to another and from one institution to another are a frequent source of patient confusion. Patient-centered care requires that those macrosystem barriers be overcome. A regional electronic health information system allowing all physicians and hospitals to instantly access any patient-sanctioned health information would be a patient-centered macrosystem improvement. Post-hospital home care, timely access to specialty referrals with immediate specialty reports back to primary care, e-prescribing that does not leave patients waiting for three days for a prescription that needs to be changed because it is not on the formulary—these and other silo-busting activities are patient centered. The Jonkoping County health system in Sweden did initiate a macrosystem improvement project based on a fictional patient named Esther. Viewing the organization of health care from Esther's perspective encouraged improvement teams to be formed with people from different clinics, hospitals, and home care services working together on Esther's behalf [35].

PATIENT-CENTERED CARE MEETS CULTURAL COMPETENCE

Patient-centered care also means being responsive to the ways in which a patient's ethnic and cultural background, socioeconomic status (including educational and literacy level), and related life situations may influence the patient's need for health care and interactions with the health care system.

Dr. Maxwell Treat was concerned. The neighborhood was changing and many patients from Vietnam had begun to seek care at his practice. As it happened, one of the two medical assistants was leaving to attend nursing school, creating an opening for a new staff member. Consulting with Vietnamese community leaders, he hired a new medical assistant whose first priority was translating for Vietnamese patients and teaching the entire practice about Vietnamese culture.

Cultural competence is "the ability of individuals to establish effective interpersonal and working relationships that supersede cultural differences" [36]. As such, cultural competence is inextricably linked with patient-centered care. Studies show that health professionals receiving cultural competence training improve their knowledge, attitudes and skills; however, evidence that this training improves health outcomes or equity of services is lacking [37]. Appendix F lists resources on cultural competence.

Language discordance between physician and patient is a major barrier to patient-centered care. Patients with limited English proficiency have more problems understanding a medical situation and have a greater risk of adverse medication reactions; access to language-concordant physicians improves but does not eliminate language barriers [38]. Quality of care is compromised if patients with limited English proficiency need but do not get interpreters. Compared with untrained interpreters and interpretation by family members, trained professional interpreters improve patient satisfaction, quality of care, and outcomes [39]. Patients are more satisfied with remote trained telephonic interpreters available from phone companies than with interpretation by untrained or family interpreters [40].

Limited English proficiency is not the only communication barrier facing many patients. About one quarter of the U.S. population has low health literacy and an additional 20% exhibits marginal health literacy. Health literacy is "the degree to which individuals have the capacity to obtain, process, and understand basic health information and services needed to make appropriate health decisions." Low health literacy is not synonymous with limited English proficiency. Many patients who are native English speakers have low health literacy, and most patients with limited English proficiency are highly literate when tested in their primary language. Most health education materials are beyond the comprehension skills of most people [41]. Compared with patients with adequate functional health literacy, those with limited health literacy report that physicians are not clear in their explanations of the patient's condition and the care they are receiving [42]. The California Health Literacy Initiative website *(www.cahealthliteracy.org)* contains a wealth of resources and materials to improve health professionals' communication with patients.

Efforts to address language, cultural, literacy, and related barriers to effective care can occur at all levels, from the individual patient-clinician relationship to the microsystem and the macrosystem. Dr. Treat's awareness of the language barriers facing his Vietnamese patients reflected sensitivity to cultural issues at the individual level, and his hiring of a Vietnamese speaking medical assistant constituted a microsystem intervention to improve cultural competence and patient-centered care. At the macrosystem level, interventions along these lines might include health plan development of, and payment for, video-based medical interpreter services.

BARRIERS TO PATIENT-CENTERED CARE

Two studies—one of adults in Massachusetts and another of Medicare beneficiaries, age 65 and above, in 13 states—suggest that patient-centered care is difficult to achieve. In 1996, 51–54% of patients surveyed gave high marks to their primary care physician for knowing their entire medical history, 36–40% said that their primary care physician knew what worried them most about their health, and 29–39% felt that the physician truly knew them as a person. Most patients gave lower rankings to other primary care clinicians who attended them when their personal physician was unavailable.

Over a 2–3-year observation period, most patient centeredness measures deteriorated. Communication between physician and patient, interpersonal treatment, and thoroughness of physical exams declined in both studies. Patient trust and access to the primary care practice declined in the Massachusetts study. Continuity and integration of care dropped for the Medicare study. Physician's knowledge of the patient was the only measure that increased slightly in both studies [43].

It is unlikely that the deterioration in patient centeredness is the fault of physicians. Rather, this trend almost certainly reflects the same system-level pressures that are creating an untenable tension between the expectations of patients and society, and what can feasibly be accomplished in primary care under existing models of practice (see Chapter 1). Both patients and clinicians are caught in the same bind, frustrated with inadequately performing systems and delivery models. Table 3–1 provides examples of how patients and clinicians can view the same problem from different perspectives. In some cases, clinician and patient appear to be in competition; in other cases, both clinician and patient are in agreement that there is insufficient time to find common ground.

The Limiting Factor of Clinician Time

Lack of time is a huge stumbling block to patient-centered care. The average patient visit is far too short to accomplish all the evidence-based care clinicians are expected to perform in addition to collaborating with patients in agenda setting, information giving, and decision making.

Preactivation and shared decision making lengthen the duration of visits. Hornberger et al. found that preactivation with a self-administered previsit questionnaire increased visit time by 34% [44]. Another study that rated the patient centeredness of visits found that the visits in the top third of ratings for patient centeredness lasted an average of 4 minutes longer than visits in the lowest third of patient centeredness scores [10]. Woolf and colleagues provide a sobering view of barriers to shared decision making [45]:

TABLE 3–1

Primary care problems viewed by physicians and patients

1. Doctor: I'm too rushed and never have time to do things right.
   Patient: I never get enough time with the doctor.

2. Doctor: It's hard to fit patients into the schedule when they need help, so they are calling and dropping in, creating more work.
   Patient: I can't get an appointment when I need it.

3. Doctor: There's never time to deal with chronic problems. Acute care always comes first.
   Patient: I wish the doctor would explain more about my diabetes.

4. Doctor: It's frustrating trying to get patients to follow my advice.
   Patient: The doctor should stop ordering me around and listen to what I have to say.

5. Doctor: I need clinical information right now, easy to get. How can people expect me to remember everything?
   Patient: I need the doctor to answer my questions with information that I can trust.

6. Doctor: I wish my office would run more smoothly. I'm tired of dealing with personnel problems.
   Patient: The office staff treats me like a number, not like a person.

7. Doctor: I'm always seeing patients of the other doctors. I want to see only my own patients.
   Patient: I have to see a different doctor for each visit.

8. Doctor: Patients are constantly calling my office for advice but no one pays us for answering the phone.
   Patient: I wish I could call my doctor to ask a few questions and save both of us a lot of time.

Today's health care system … clings to an outdated model—relying on busy clinicians to keep their patients informed—a holdover from an earlier time when a physician's impromptu advice was sufficient and when there was little concern about its inherent incompleteness or bias … Current reimbursement incentives reward costly procedures and rushed visits; they discourage the counseling that ensures that procedures are warranted in the first place and that gives patients the self-management tools on which the effectiveness of those treatments often depends.

Clinician time is also a rate-limiting step in ensuring timely access to care—a key element of patient-centered care. Because many primary care clinicians have too many patients in their panels, demand for visits often exceeds the capacity to provide appointments, making timely access impossible (see Chapter 6).

One *win-win* strategy, to creating practices that can be at once more patient centered and more satisfying work environments for clinicians and staff, is to pursue the innovative new models of care introduced in Chapter 2. To make primary care more patient centered, the answer is not, *make clinicians work harder and longer.* Solutions lie in harnessing team members and electronic technology in redesigned office processes that optimize the efficient role of the primary care clinician in a well-functioning microsystem.

In addition, just as clinicians and patients attempt to develop a partnership, so can practices forge partnerships with their patients. Because practice patterns, convenient to patients, may not always be feasible for physicians and practice staff, dialogue within the microsystem between patients and the practice is key to fostering patient centeredness. The United Kingdom has launched citizens' groups to advise medical facilities on policy issues [46]. Patient-centered U.S. primary care practices could do the same. Moreover, practices can initiate periodic patient satisfaction surveys (see Appendix D) that ask specific questions rather than the relatively meaningless single question: *Are you satisfied with your care?*

CONCLUSION: PATIENT-CENTERED CARE IS A PARTNERSHIP

Patient-centered care is a partnership between patients, caregivers, clinical practices, and the health care system. In the realm of the patient-clinician encounter, patient-centered care involves the seeking of common ground between patient preference and evidence-based medicine. In the domain of the primary care microsystem, patient-centered care involves clinical and administrative processes that best meet patient needs while preserving the practice's financial viability and morale of the clinical team. In the outermost orbit of the health care macrosystem, patient-centered care refers to a health care system organized to promote access to care for the entire population and to coordinate services in a seamless manner, balanced by the resource constraints under which the macrosystem operates.

Patient-centered care remains a needed counterweight to the flawed reality of many patient-clinician encounters, and to the difficulties patients experience accessing primary care and navigating the larger health system. But patient-centered care, in its essence, is about partnerships.

REFERENCES

1. Institute of Medicine: *Crossing the Quality Chasm: A New Health System for the 21st Century*. Washington, DC, National Academy Press, 2001.
2. Future of Family Medicine Project Leadership Committee: The future of family medicine. Ann Fam Med. 2004;2(Suppl 1):S3–S32.
3. Society of General Internal Medicine: The Future of General Internal Medicine. 2003. (*www.sgim.org/futureofGIMreport.cfm*)
4. American College of Physicians: *Patient-Centered, Physician-Guided Care for the Chronically Ill: The American College of Physicians Prescription for Change*. Philadelphia, PA, American College of Physicians, 2005.
5. Little P, Everitt H, Williamson I, et al: Preferences of patients for patient centered approach to consultation in primary care. BMJ. 2001;322:468–472.
6. Swenson SL, Buell S, Zettler P, et al: Patient-centered communication: do patients really prefer it? J Gen Intern Med. 2004;19:1069–1079.
7. Deber RB, Kraetschmer N, Irvine J: What role do patients wish to play in treatment decision making? Arch Intern Med. 1996;156:1414–1420.
8. Frosch DL, Kaplan RM: Shared decision making in clinical medicine: past research and future directions. Am J Prev Med. 1999;17:285–294.
9. Stewart M, Brown JB, Donner A, et al: The impact of patient-centered care on outcomes. J Fam Pract. 2000;49:796–804
10. Epstein RM, Franks P, Shields CG, et al: Patient-centered communication and diagnostic testing. Ann Fam Med. 2005;3:415–421.
11. Coulter A: What do patients and the public want from primary care? BMJ. 2005;331:1199–1201.
12. Schoen C, Osborn R, Huynh PT, et al: Primary care and health system performance: adults' experiences in five countries. Health Aff Web Exclusive. October 28, 2004;W4-487–503.
13. Mead N, Bower P: Patient-centeredness: a conceptual framework and review of the empirical literature. Soc Sci Med. 2000;51:1087–1110.
14. Marvel MK, Epstein RM, Flowers K, et al: Soliciting the patient's agenda. JAMA. 1999;281:283–287.
15. Beckman HB, Frankel RM: The effect of physician behavior on the collection of data. Ann Intern Med. 1984;101:692–696.
16. Deyo RA, Diehl AK: Patient satisfaction with medical care for low back pain. Spine. 1986;11:28–30.
17. Roter DL, Hall JA: Studies of doctor-patient interaction. Annu Rev Public Health. 1989;10:163–180.
18. Waitzkin H: Doctor-patient communication: clinical implications of social scientific research. JAMA. 1984;252:2441–2446.
19. Svarstad B: Physician-Patient Communication and Patient Conformity with Medical Advice. In D. Mechanic ed: *The Growth of Bureaucratic Medicine*. New York: Wiley,1976.

20. Hulka BS, Kupper LL, Cassel JC, et al: Doctor-patient communication and outcomes among diabetic patients. J Health Commun. 1975;1(1):15–27.
21. Schillinger D, Machtinger E, Wang F, et al: Preventing Medication Errors in Ambulatory Care: The Importance of Establishing Regimen Concordance Advances in Patient Safety: From Research to Implementation. Volume 1. Research findings. Rockville, MD: Agency for Healthcare Research and Quality, 2005.
22. Stewart AL, Napoles-Springer A, Perez-Stable EJ, et al: Interpersonal processes of care in diverse populations. Milbank Q. 1999;77:305–339.
23. Schillinger D, Piette J, Grumbach K, et al: Closing the loop. Physician communication with diabetic patients who have low health literacy. Arch Intern Med. 2003;163:83–90.
24. Braddock CH, Edwards KA, Hasenberg NM, et al: Informed decision making in outpatient practice. JAMA. 1999;282:2313–2320.
25. Cooper LA, Roter DL, Johnson RL, et al: Patient-centered communication, ratings of care, and concordance of patient and physician race. Ann Intern Med. 2003;139:907–915.
26. Greenfield S, Kaplan S, Ware JE: Expanding patient involvement in care. Ann Intern Med. 1985;102:520–528.
27. Cegala DJ, Marinelli T, Post D: The effects of patient communication skills training on compliance. Arch Fam Med. 2000:9:57–64.
28. Cegala DJ, McClure L, Marinelli TM, et al: The effects of communication skills training on patients' participation during medical interviews. Patient Educ Couns. 2000;41:209–222.
29. Greenfield S, Kaplan SH, Ware JE, et al: Patients' participation in medical care. J Gen Intern Med. 1988;3:448–457.
30. Roter DL: Patient question asking in physician-patient interaction. Health Psychol. 1984;3:395–409.
31. Roter DL. Patient participation in the patient-provider interaction. Health Educ Monogr. 1997;5:281–315.
32. O'Connor AM, Llewellyn-Thomas HA, Flood AB: Modifying unwarranted variations in health care: shared decision making using patient decision aids. Health Aff Web Exclusive. October 7, 2004;VAR 63–72.
33. Schillinger D, Villela T, Saba G: Creating a context for effective intervention in the clinical care of vulnerable patients. In King T, Wheeler M, Bindman A, et al eds: *Medical Management of Vulnerable and Underserved Patients: Principles, Practice and Populations.* New York, McGraw-Hill; 2006.
34. Saba GW, Wong ST, Schillinger D, et al: Shared decision making and the experience of partnership in primary care. Ann Fam Med. 2006;4:54–62.
35. (*www.ihi.org/IHI/Topics/Flow/PatientFlow/ImprovementStories/ImprovingPatient FlowTheEstherProjectinSweden.htm*)
36. Cooper LA, Roter DL: Patient-provider communication: The effect of race and ethnicity on process and outcomes of healthcare. In: Smedley BD, Stith

AY, Nelson AR, eds: *Unequal Treatment: Confronting Racial and Ethnic Disparities in Healthcare.* Washington, DC: The National Academies Press; 2002:552–593.

37. Beach MC, Price EG, Gary TL, et al: Cultural competence. Med Care. 2005;43:356–373.
38. Wilson E, Chen AH, Grumbach K, et al: Effects of limited English proficiency and physician language on health care comprehension. J Gen Intern Med. 2005;20:800–806.
39. Flores G: The impact of medical interpreter services on the quality of health care: a systematic review. Med Care Res Rev. 2005;62(3):255–299.
40. Lee LJ, Batal HA, Maselli, JH, et al: Effect of Spanish interpretation method on patient satisfaction in an urban walk-in clinic. J Gen Intern Med. 2002;17:641–645.
41. Paasche-Orlow MK, Parker RM, Gazmararian JA, et al: The prevalence of limited health literacy. J Gen Intern Med. 2005;20:175–184.
42. Schillinger D, Bindman A, Wang F, et al: Functional health literacy and the quality of physician-patient communication among diabetes patients. Patient Educ Couns. 2004;52:315–323.
43. Safran DG: Primary care performance: views from the patient. In Showstack J, Rothman AA, Hassmiller SB, eds: *The Future of Primary Care.* San Francisco, CA, Jossey-Bass:2004.
44. Hornberger J, Thom D, Macurdy T: Effects of a self-administered previsit questionnaire to enhance awareness of patients' concerns in primary care. J Gen Intern Med. 1997;12:597–606.
45. Woolf SH, Chan ECY, Harris R, et al: Promoting informed choice: transforming health care to dispense knowledge for decision making. Ann Intern Med. 2005;143:293–300.
46. Gold MR: Tea, biscuits, and health care prioritizing. Health Aff. 2005;24(1):234–239.

Improving Primary Care for Patients with Chronic Illness

Randall Short, a 64-year-old patient with diabetes, comes for his 15-minute visit with Dr. Ron Madden. After evaluating Mr. Short's acutely painful knee and treating his gastroesophageal reflux disease, Dr. Madden has 3 minutes left to assess diabetic control. Having fruitlessly searched through Mr. Short's medical records to find the last eye examination results and hemoglobin A1c (Hb A1c) and lipid levels, Dr. Madden gives up in frustration and schedules another visit during his day off to manage Mr. Short's diabetes. Mr. Short was never taught how to check his sugars at home.

Juanita Feliz arrives for her planned diabetes-management visit. At a previous acute care visit, she discussed her knee pain and esophageal reflux with Dr. Lisa Newman. Ms. Feliz, as taught in her self-management class, hands her home glucose record to the medical assistant, who scans it into the electronic medical record, reviews with Ms. Feliz the reminder pop-up message, refers her for an eye examination and test of urine microalbumin, and prints for Ms. Feliz and Dr. Newman a graph showing the last 2 years of her Hb A1c (normal) and low-density lipoprotein cholesterol (LDL-C) (elevated) results. Dr. Newman briefly discusses with Ms. Feliz an action plan to address hyperlipidemia and arranges two visits: one to the pharmacist, who adjusts Ms. Feliz's medication doses according to a practice guideline–based protocol, and another to the nutritionist to discuss low-fat diet options.

One hundred million persons in the United States have at least one chronic condition. Half of these individuals have more than one chronic illness. Eighty-eight percent of people aged 65 years or older have one or more chronic illnesses, and one-quarter of these have four or more conditions. Chronic illness accounts for three-quarters of total national health care expenditures [1, 2].

Most patients with chronic conditions are managed in primary care. However, the majority of patients with hypertension [3], diabetes [4], tobacco addiction [5], congestive heart failure (CHF) [6], chronic atrial fibrillation [7], asthma [8], and depression [9] are inadequately treated (see Chapter 1). Why is primary care unable to provide consistent high quality for people with these common health problems?

Frequently, the acute symptoms and concerns of the patient crowd out the less urgent need to bring chronic illness under optimal management. Edward Wagner has called this phenomenon *the tyranny of the urgent* [10]. Clinicians—as in the vignette describing Dr. Madden—routinely experience the lack of time to handle acute, chronic, and preventive care. Quantifying this problem, Ostbye and associates found that for a typical panel of 2500 patients, it would take 10.6 hours per day for a physician to provide good management of common chronic conditions [11]. A companion study found that for a similar panel, preventive services would consume another 7.4 hours per day [12].

The current organization of primary care practice, which makes physicians responsible for acute, chronic, and preventive care, is unsustainable. Visits are brief and little planning takes place to ensure that acute, chronic, and preventive needs are all addressed. Lacking is a division of labor that would allow nonphysician personnel to take greater responsibility in chronic care management. Too often, caring for chronic illness features an uninformed, passive patient interacting with an unprepared practice team, resulting in frustrating, inadequate encounters [10].

THE CHRONIC CARE MODEL

Edward Wagner and associates at the MacColl Institute for Healthcare Innovation—affiliated with Group Health Cooperative of Puget Sound in Seattle, Washington—have developed a model for primary care of patients with chronic illness. The Chronic Care Model, a guide to be used in developing effective chronic care, does not offer a quick and easy fix; it is a multidimensional solution to a complex problem [13–15]. The Chronic Care Model constitutes a major rethinking of primary care practice, as pictured in the opening vignette about Dr. Newman.

Chronic care takes place within three overlapping galaxies: (1) the entire community, with its myriad resources and numerous public and private policies; (2) the health care system, including its payment structures; and (3) the provider organization, whether an integrated delivery system, a small clinic, or a loose network of physician practices.

Within this trigalactic universe, the workings of which may help or hinder optimal chronic care, the Chronic Care Model identifies six essential elements: community resources and policies, health care organization, self-management support, delivery system design, decision support, and clinical information systems (Figure 4–1). What are these six pillars of the chronic care edifice?

Community Resources and Policies

To improve chronic care, provider organizations need linkages with community-based resources, for example, exercise programs, senior centers, and self-help groups. Community linkages—for example, with hospitals

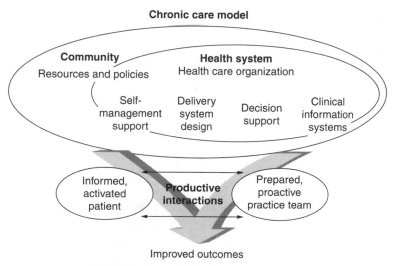

FIGURE 4–1. The Chronic Care Model.

offering patient education classes or home care agencies providing case managers—are especially helpful for small physician offices with limited resources.

Health Care Organization

The structure, goals, and values of a provider organization and its relationships with purchasers, insurers, and other providers form the foundation upon which the remaining four components of the Chronic Care Model rest. If an organization's goals and leaders do not view chronic care as a priority, innovation will not take place. The reimbursement environment of a provider organization has a major impact on chronic care improvements, which are more likely to survive throughout the long term if they increase revenues or reduce expenses. If purchasers and insurers fail to reward chronic care quality, improvements are difficult to sustain.

Self-Management Support

For chronic conditions, patients themselves become the principal caregivers. People live with chronic illness for many years; management of these illnesses can be taught to most patients, and substantial segments of that management—diet, exercise, self-measurement (e.g., using glucometers or bathroom scales), and medication use—are under the direct control of the patient. Self-management support involves collaboratively helping patients and their families acquire the skills and confidence to manage their chronic illness; providing self-management tools (e.g., blood pressure cuffs, glucometers, diets, and referrals to community resources); and routinely assessing problems and accomplishments. This component of the Chronic Care Model is discussed at length in Chapter 5.

Delivery System Design

Delivery system design involves three components: the formation of primary care teams, case management (also called care management), and planned chronic care visits. The essential element of delivery system redesign is planned care, which includes all three of these components.

Planned care is any encounter with a patient or group of patients at which there is only one agenda item—the management of patients' chronic condition(s). Planned care combats the *tyranny of the urgent* by separating chronic from acute care visits. Planned care can take place in individual or group visits, by telephone, at home, by e-mail, or Internet (see Chapter 7). It can be conducted by physicians, nonphysician clinicians, nurses, pharmacists, health educators, nutritionists, community health workers/promotoras, or trained patients.

The scope of a planned visit varies depending on the competencies of the person leading the visit. Visits led by physicians, nonphysician clinicians, nurses, or pharmacists can include patient education; self-management support; referral to laboratory studies, specialists or community resources; interpretation of laboratory results; and medication management. Visits led by other caregivers tend to focus on patient education, self-management support, referrals, and interpretation of laboratory results, but do not generally provide medication management.

Case or care management is a type of planned visit. Case management is an older term, which tended to involve the matching of patients with the most appropriate, and often the lowest cost, level of care. Care management, generally performed by nurses, pharmacists, health educators, nutritionists, and (for asthma) respiratory therapists, is a newer term that emphasizes direct clinical care by the care manager.

Planned care is frequently provided by nonphysician caregivers because visits with physicians may turn into multiagenda acute and chronic visits, thereby subverting the intent of a single-agenda encounter. It is easier to separate chronic from acute care if other caregivers provide planned chronic care. For that reason, multidisciplinary teams are needed to conduct planned care.

Because self-management support requires caregivers spending considerable time with patients until the patients become successful self-managers, it cannot be properly implemented without planned visits.

Decision Support

Evidence-based clinical practice guidelines provide standards for optimal chronic care. Ideally, specialist expertise is a mere telephone call away and does not always require full specialty referral. Guidelines are reinforced by physician *champions* leading educational sessions for practice teams.

Clinical Information Systems

Clinical information systems have three important roles:

1. Registries are lists of all patients with a particular chronic condition on an organization or physician's panel and include important clinical data regarding that condition [16]. Take the example of diabetes. Data for patients with a diabetes-related diagnosis code, diabetic prescription, or laboratory test result indicating diabetes are entered electronically into the diabetic registry. Laboratory values—Hb A1c, LDL-C, and urine microalbumin—automatically flow to the registry. Ideally, eye and foot examinations and blood pressure measurements are also entered. The registry may feed into a reminder pop-up message on the electronic medical record, which flags laboratory work or examinations not performed according to schedule. With paper charts, reminder sheets can be printed for each visit by the diabetic patient. As a population tool, registry data can be electronically sorted to identify and contact patients with elevated Hb A1c levels or those lacking up-to-date eye examination results.

2. Reminders help primary care teams comply with practice guidelines. Reminder systems may involve placing a sheet of paper on the front of a chart, reminding the care team that preventive or chronic care actions are needed, or may be done through *pop-ups* on an electronic medical record.

3. Feedback to physicians shows how each is performing on chronic illness measures. Data collected from registries or chart audits can be fed back to physicians to inform them of their performance compared with their peers. Examples of measures fed back to physicians include the percent of diabetics on the physician's panel with Hb A1c levels below 8, or the percent of persistent asthmatics using steroid inhalers.

The Interdependence of Chronic Care Model Components

The six components of the Chronic Care Model are interdependent, building upon one another [17]. Community resources—for example, exercise programs and peer support groups—help patients acquire self-management skills. Delivery system redesign, the formation of primary care teams with a division of labor, is essential to teach self-management because physicians do not have the time and may not be properly trained for this activity. For chronic disease registries to be successful, redesigning delivery systems is necessary so that one member of a primary care team is responsible for working the registry. Clinical practice guidelines, a key decision-support tool, provide the evidence upon which physician feedback data and reminder systems are based. Chronic Care Model elements are unlikely to be introduced or maintained without an organizational environment featuring innovative leadership and favorable finances.

As its ultimate goal, the Chronic Care Model envisions an informed, activated patient interacting with a prepared, proactive practice team, resulting in high quality, satisfying encounters and improved outcomes.

The Chronic Care Model and Prevention

The Chronic Care Model is also a useful construct for improving clinical preventive services, including both cancer screening and counseling for healthy behavior change [18]. Chronic care and preventive care overlap because secondary prevention (interventions targeted to people with a chronic condition designed to reverse or retard the condition from progressing) and chronic care are essentially the same thing.

IMPLEMENTING THE CHRONIC CARE MODEL

Jill Goode (RN) was frustrated. She knew the kids with asthma at Lo-Budget Family Health Center were not getting the care they needed. Seeing 30 patients a day, the doctors were just too busy and Ms. Goode spent all day triaging phone calls to make sure that people with urgent problems could be seen promptly. The federal Bureau of Primary Health Care, which provided some funding to her health center, sent out an invitation to join something called a collaborative to improve the care of childhood asthma. Ms. Goode persuaded the center director to send a team of a physician, nurse, and medical assistant.

The collaborative's first learning session was a wake-up call. Someone from the Institute for Healthcare Improvement (IHI) talked about the

Improvement Model—how to make changes in a medical practice. Dr. Edward Wagner explained the Chronic Care Model, which confirmed Ms. Goode's impression that high-quality chronic care required systematic changes in primary care practice. All 20 teams, from health centers around the country, learned how to set up registries to track asthma care. The teams were told that they had to report their performance to the collaborative faculty every month. When they returned to Lo-Budget Family Health Center they were energized, but nervous about how the rest of the center would react.

Is the Chronic Care Model a utopian concept, impossible to implement in the rough-and-tumble world of primary care? The model is not an abstract theory but a concrete guide to improving practice. A list of resources on improving chronic care and a survey to evaluate patients' experiences in receiving chronic care are available in Appendices J and K.

Many organizations have attempted to introduce the Chronic Care Model, often inspired by national learning collaboratives. Some have enjoyed success. Others succeeded but were unable to sustain the improvements. The case studies presented here involve private medical practices, two integrated delivery systems, and a community health center.

Premier Health Partners

In 1998, Premier Health Partners joined a diabetes collaborative led by IHI and the Improving Chronic Illness Care (ICIC) project directed by Edward Wagner. Located in Dayton, Ohio, Premier Health Partners is a health system based on the traditional private practice model. One hundred physicians working in 36 private offices make up Premier's primary physician network. Starting with one physician and gradually adding all primary care practices, Premier used the Chronic Care Model to improve diabetes care. By 2001, for the entire primary care network, the proportion of diabetic patients with Hb A1c levels below 7% had risen from 42% to 70%. Similar improvements were recorded for foot examination results, urine microalbumin levels, and use of angiotensin-converting enzyme inhibitors.

Decision support is provided through practice guidelines, academic detailing, and a toolkit of printed materials that incorporate practice guidelines into the day-to-day care of diabetic patients. Self-management support includes individual and group classes and flowcharts on which patients record their own laboratory test results. Delivery system redesign began with the development of practice teams in which physicians and nurses work together to monitor diabetes flow sheets. Premier Health

Partners has achieved its improved diabetes care with a rudimentary but effective information system—medical-record reviews in each primary care practice generate physician-specific data on diabetes measures that are circulated, unblinded to all physicians. These data have stimulated physicians with poor performance to improve.

HealthPartners Medical Group

HealthPartners Medical Group (HPMG), an integrated delivery system based in Minneapolis, Minnesota, began a diabetes registry in 1994, promulgated diabetes guidelines in 1997, and began to feed back diabetes-related clinical data to clinicians in 1997. The registry provides each physician with a quarterly at-risk list that prioritizes patients according to Hb A1c and LDL-C levels and presence of coronary artery disease. These quarterly reports also provide graphs showing physician and clinic performance on Hb A1c and LDL-C measures. Clinician reminder prompts have also been utilized. Clinician training on diabetes was conducted, starting in 1999, and clinician *pay-for-performance* financial incentives were launched in 2002. Patient self-management training is performed in planned visits by diabetes nurses. Case management is available for patients designated by the at-risk list to require more intensive management. HPMG has thus instituted the major components of the Chronic Care Model. From 1994 to 2003, the average Hb A1c level for HPMG adults with diabetes declined from 8.3 to 6.9. Average LDL-C levels for these patients dropped from 132 to 97 during these years [19].

Clinica Campesina

More than 700 community health centers operate in the United States, serving 9.6 million patients at thousands of sites. Community health centers operate with funds from the federal Bureau of Primary Health Care, Medicare, Medicaid, and state health departments. Eighty-six percent of community health center patients live below 200% of the federal poverty line, 40% are uninsured, and 64% are ethnic minorities who experience higher-than-average rates of chronic illness.

In 1998, the Bureau of Primary Health Care initiated the Health Disparities Initiative, a concerted program aimed at eliminating racial, ethnic, and socioeconomic disparities [20]. The Bureau funded a full-time coordinator in each of five geographic clusters, and one community health center from each cluster was picked as the lead organization. The five coordinators and a team from each of the five lead community health centers attended ICIC-IHI's training sessions on organizational change and care of chronic illness. By 2001, diabetes improvement programs had spread from 5 to 200 clinical sites; in 2002, 371 community health centers had chronic care projects for diabetes, cardiovascular disease, asthma, depression, or all four. A leader in the initial diabetes collaborative was Clinica Campesina Family Health Services.

Clinica Campesina provides care to a largely uninsured Hispanic population around Denver, Colorado. Assisted by the diabetes collaborative, Clinica Campesina implemented most components of the Chronic Care Model, including primary care teams with a division of labor, a diabetes registry (using a rudimentary information system requiring clinic staff to input data), physician reminders, diabetes group visits (delivery system redesign), and activation of patients to manage their illness through diabetes education and collaborative setting of diabetes treatment goals during each clinic visit. Patients are provided with self-management plans allowing them to choose self-improvement goals such as walking a mile each day or stopping tobacco use. Monthly printouts of the registry are distributed to all physicians, and to relieve physicians' workload, medical assistants read patients' flow sheets and make appropriate preparations for needed examinations or tests. Outreach is provided to patients on the registry who have poorly controlled illness or difficulty coming to the clinic.

Clinica Campesina's self-reported data show that the average Hb A1c level of its diabetic population dropped from 10.5% in October 1998 to 8.6% in March 2000. The percentage of diabetic patients with at least two Hb A1c tests within a year rose from 11% in October 1998 to 71% in June 2000. The percentage of diabetic patients with self-management goals jumped from 3% in February 1999 to 65% in March 2000. The percentage of those having eye examinations climbed from 7% to 51%, and the percentage having foot examinations rose from 15% to 76% in the same period.

Kaiser-Permanente Northern California

Kaiser Health Plan and the associated Permanente Medical Group serve 3 million people in the northern California region. Within Kaiser-Permanente Northern California (KPNC), 22% of adult enrollees, mainly those with chronic conditions, generate 47% of adult ambulatory visits and 74% of nonobstetric hospital days. By 1999, KPNC had launched

Chronic Care Management programs targeting diabetes, coronary artery disease, hyperlipidemia, asthma, and CHF. Kaiser-Permanente Northern California invested millions of dollars in these programs, hoping to improve health outcomes and thereby create savings through fewer hospitalizations and emergency department visits. From 1996 to 2002, quality indicators for coronary heart disease, CHF, diabetes, and asthma showed substantial improvements [21].

Chronic Care Management divides KPNC's chronic condition population of 400,000 into three levels. Patients at level 1 have their chronic condition under reasonable control and receive care through their primary care team. Patients at level 2 have poorly controlled conditions, for example, diabetic patients with Hb A1c levels above 10% qualify for level 2. Level 3 is composed of patients with complex multidiagnoses, high-use patients, or both who receive case management by registered nurses or medical social workers within the primary care team; because patients have multiple diagnoses, level 3 case management is not disease specific.

The most far-reaching delivery system redesign involves level 2 patients, who are referred to disease-specific care managers who may be attached to a primary care team. Care managers—nurses, health educators, pharmacists, respiratory therapists, or dietitians—exist for management of diabetes, hyperlipidemia, asthma, and CHF. They are responsible for a list of patients with whom they work intensively for a 6- to 15-month period, after which, if the illness is better controlled, the patient returns to level 1. Care managers, who attend training programs, update seminars, and peer group meetings, are mentored by disease-specific physician champions.

Adult asthma provides an example of how KPNC's Chronic Care Management programs operate. Data for asthmatic adults are electronically entered into the asthma registry according to diagnosis code or use of asthma medications. Patients with an asthma-related emergency department visit, hospitalization, or pharmacy data revealing two prednisone bursts or an excess of asthma inhalers are designated as level 2 or high risk and referred to an asthma care manager. Care managers—nurses, respiratory therapists, or pharmacists—arrange a personal visit, including patient self-management support with training on use of inhalers, spacers, and peak flow meters. Care managers can change medications according to clinical protocols. Patients are taught about triggers and environmental controls and how to stage the severity of their illness. Care managers help patients set specific monthly goals, for example, regular use of steroid inhalers or keeping the cat off the bed at night. Smokers are referred to smoking cessation classes.

Chronic Care Management leaders are concerned about level 1, which handles 85–90% of KPNC's chronic care patients (only 12% of asthmatic patients are in level 2 at any given time). Even if level 2 is working well, failure to improve level 1 care threatens population-wide improvement in performance measures. To remedy this problem, the asthma program is planning training sessions for health educators on primary care teams, physician-specific feedback, and prompts reminding physicians to check peak flows, assess asthma symptoms, review self-management care plans, and improve medication use.

The clinical information system tracks the asthma-inhaled medication ratio (anti-inflammatory canisters divided by anti-inflammatory plus bronchodilator canisters). The long-term goal (benchmark) for this ratio is for 95% of primary care physicians to have a ratio higher than 0.3. From 1998 to early 2001, according to KPNC's own data, the percentage exceeding 0.3 increased from 52% to 79% (32% have a ratio greater than 0.5).

The information system also tracks the percentage of asthma patients at high risk of an acute event (those with a recent emergency department visit, hospitalization, or high volume of asthma-related prescriptions). This measure dropped from 13.5% in 1998 to 9.1% in early 2001, with the best medical center reporting a rate of 6.5%. The long-term benchmark is 8%. From 1996 to 2000, the emergency department visit rate declined from 10 per 100 persistent asthmatic patients to 4. Through registry-generated data, KPNC determines which of its 17 medical centers are performing well and can provide assistance to centers with less adequate performance.

These case studies illustrate how a broad variety of practice organizations have implemented the Chronic Care Model at the primary care level. In each case, the organizations are attempting to transform primary care practice from the untenable situation faced by Dr. Madden in the opening vignette to the idealized world inhabited by Dr. Newman. None of the organizations has achieved full implementation of the Chronic Care Model, but all have made important strides toward that goal.

DO CHRONIC CARE MODEL COMPONENTS IMPROVE CLINICAL OUTCOMES?

Dr. Bob Lerner was upset. The nurse, Jill Goode, at the health center where he worked, had come back from some meeting called a collaborative and was telling the doctors that they needed to improve their care of patients with asthma. Dr. Lerner worked hard and did a fine job; he didn't appreciate that kind of criticism. When the initial data from the new asthma registry was distributed, only 45% of his patients with persistent asthma were on controller medications.

"The problem," argued Dr. Lerner, "is patient noncompliance. The patients aren't picking up the controller medications I am prescribing." Ms. Goode was not convinced. "Since you don't send your patients to the health educator, how much time have you spent teaching patients about the different kinds of medications they need to improve their asthma?" Dr. Lerner said he would cooperate with the asthma improvement project for 1 month and if he saw no results, he would organize the other physicians to close down the project. A month later, when the registry data showed significant improvement in asthma control, Dr. Lerner spoke at the doctors' meeting cautiously praising the asthma initiative. He went to the collaborative's second learning session where Dr. Ed Wagner presented evidence from the literature showing that the Chronic Care Model could improve asthma care. Dr. Lerner was highly impressed and became a physician champion of chronic care improvement.

Many studies have examined the impact of Chronic Care Model components on processes of care, clinical outcomes, and costs for a number of chronic diseases. These studies, including references, are reviewed in Appendix N for three of the four Chronic Care Model components internal to a primary care practice—decision support, delivery system redesign, and clinical information systems. The fourth internal component—self-management support—is discussed in Chapter 5. A brief summary is presented here.

Decision Support

Simply making clinical practice guidelines available to physicians does not change medical practice. Traditional continuing medical education conferences are also not effective, while academic detailing (outreach visits by physician educators) and the influence of local opinion leaders are usually successful. Combining several educational interventions produces a greater proportion of positive changes in health outcomes than using a single intervention.

Delivery System Redesign

The key element of delivery system redesign is planned care. Ample evidence demonstrates that planned care—whether in individual or group visits—is associated with improved processes of care and/or clinical outcomes in diabetes, hypertension, coronary heart disease, CHF, asthma, and anti-coagulation, depression, and chronic disease in general. The literature review is available in Appendix N.

Clinical Information Systems

Reminder prompts are usually effective in improving care, apparently working better than physician feedback, which has been found to be helpful only in some studies. Registries by themselves have no impact, but when used as a substrate for reminders, feedback, and tracking entire populations of patients, they are very effective.

Multiple Chronic Care Model Component Interventions

A review of 39 studies of Chronic Care Model components to improve the care of patients with diabetes found improvements in the process or outcomes of care in 32 studies. All five of the studies featuring all four of the internal Chronic Care Model components had a positive result, but it could not be determined whether a greater number of components were associated with a greater effect. It was impressive that 19 of the 20 interventions including a self-management support component improved a process or outcome of care [15]. Most reviews of a mixture of Chronic Care Model components have shown improvement in care processes and/or clinical outcomes.

DOES THE CHRONIC CARE MODEL SAVE MONEY?

Dr. Michael Herz, a cardiologist at Bottom-Line Hospital specializing in heart failure, started a program using nurses to visit and make telephone calls to heart failure patients in their homes. The nurses trained patients to reduce their salt intake, to weigh themselves daily, and to increase their diuretic doses if the weight increased by more than 3 pounds. The nurses also assisted patients in taking their medications properly. After a year, the patients in Dr. Herz's program felt better and had reduced their heart failure hospital admissions by 50%, compared with patients receiving *standard care. The day that Dr. Herz's study was published in a major medical journal, Bottom-Line Hospital's CEO came to his office. "Michael, I'm sorry but we are closing down your heart failure program. By reducing admissions, the program lost the hospital $500,000 last year."*

Does implementation of Chronic Care Model components save health care dollars? There are several viewpoints: (1) It does reduce costs, (2) It does not reduce costs, or (3) Nobody knows. A more reasonable perspective is—it depends.

It depends on: What chronic condition? Which patients with that chronic condition? What kind of health care institution and how is that institution reimbursed?

Which Patients with Which Chronic Conditions?

Evidence from several systematic reviews of controlled trials is extremely strong that health care costs can be substantially reduced by implementing post-hospital programs for some patients with CHF [22–24]. Because CHF is so common and so costly, with a huge rate of readmission shortly following hospital discharge, the potential for major money savings is great. The cost-saving programs focus on CHF patients who are hospitalized and at high risk (due to severe disease or poor social support) for recurrent hospital admissions or emergency department (ED) visits. The programs that are effective in reducing readmissions and ED visits: (1) begin prior to discharge and continue immediately after discharge, and (2) are generally managed by nurse care managers who keep a close track of patients' weight and medication adherence not only by telephone but also with face-to-face visits [25].

Substantial evidence also finds that cost savings are possible for adults and children with moderate or severe (not mild) asthma who have a history of asthma-related hospitalizations or recurrent emergency department visits [15]; these findings also apply to patients in Medicaid programs [15, 26].

For other conditions, such as diabetes, hypertension, coronary heart disease, and depression, persuasive evidence that costs can be reduced is lacking. Some studies demonstrate cost savings for diabetes [15] and for secondary prevention of coronary heart disease [27, 28]. Disease management vendor companies claim to have reduced costs through programs for people with diabetes who are at high risk for expensive complications [29], but other reports question these findings [21, 30].

Although the introduction of Chronic Care Model components at Northern California's Kaiser Permanente system did not reduce health care costs, those innovations were implemented in a system that already had relatively low costs and low hospitalization rates prior to the innovations [21, 31].

A meta-analysis of chronic care costs was published in 2005. Pooling data from 67 studies of a wide variety of chronic disease management programs, including heart disease, diabetes, and asthma, the author found that disease management does reduce costs for all three conditions, and that the cost reductions are greater for patients with more severe disease. The savings, which were small or moderate in size, were mainly the result of an average 25% drop in hospitalization rates for patients receiving disease management interventions [32].

Reimbursement and Savings from Improved Chronic Care

Top-of-the-Line Hospital, owned by an integrated delivery system that receives all its income through capitation payments, instituted a CHF program with primary care–based nurse care managers calling patients in their homes to monitor diets, weights, and use of medications. Hospitalization rates for these patients fell dramatically, thereby reducing the hospital's expenses, improving its financial position, and demonstrating the economic value of primary care.

Bottom-Line Hospital, which receives diagnosis-related group payments for Medicare patients, attempted a similar CHF program that also reduced hospital admissions. However, the reduced admissions meant fewer Medicare dollars, causing the hospital to lose money on the program. The program was discontinued.

For the Chronic Care Model to be widely and permanently implemented, there needs to be a business case for chronic care: Does better chronic care improve the financial bottom line? For whom does it improve the bottom line?

The cost savings achievable through improvements in CHF and asthma result from fewer days in the hospital and less use of the emergency department. Whether these savings translate into a favorable business case depends entirely on how the hospital is paid, as the preceding vignettes demonstrate. If the hospital is reimbursed by capitation or is part of a capitated integrated system, reduced hospital and ED use can save money for the organization. The incentives are aligned to produce a business case for chronic care.

If, in contrast, the innovating hospital or integrated system is reimbursed per diem or fee-for-service, fewer days in the hospital and fewer ED visits translate into a loss of revenue. Under Medicare's diagnosis-related group system, fewer hospital admissions reduce revenue. Doing the right thing loses money for the institution, and the business case for improving chronic care evaporates. Under per diem, fee-for-service, or diagnosis-related group payment to hospitals and integrated systems, the insurer (whether Medicare, Medicaid, HMO, preferred provider organization, or self-insured employer), not the organization paying for the improvements, may save money from improved chronic care. In these cases, insurers, who reap the benefits, should be paying for chronic care improvement programs.

For a primary care practice, fee-for-service payment may be compatible with a favorable business case for chronic care. The use of registries and reminder systems may increase the number of physician visits, laboratory tests, and billable patient education sessions, resulting in higher fee-for-service revenues. However, the planned care encounters that are central to improved chronic care are often performed by caregivers who are not reimbursed for their time; in addition, phone and electronic encounters are often not paid for. Overall, current payment practices do not encourage primary care practices to implement the Chronic Care Model.

Because so much chronic illness is concentrated in the elderly population, one important option for creating a positive business case is Medicare reform. Medicare's payment methods are often copied by private insurers and, because Medicare is such a large program, can change the behavior of primary care practices. It is possible that Medicare will institute a pay-for-performance system, rewarding practices that improve chronic care performance measures. However, this reform is not sufficient. Medicare needs to pay for chronic care start-up costs (including information systems) and reimburse nonphysician personnel who provide planned care.

In summary, the *business case* for better chronic care depends on many factors. The pessimistic view was expressed by one California physician, "Hospitals make more money cutting off a diabetic foot than providing good diabetes management." An optimistic view holds that good care up front avoids expensive care to handle complications; the business case based on that view only applies to some patients with some conditions in some institutions, but is by no means a universal truth.

CHANGING PRIMARY CARE TO INCORPORATE
THE CHRONIC CARE MODEL

The Chronic Care Model is complicated. Is it feasible to integrate all six components of the model into a busy primary care practice?

Although adoption of the entire Chronic Care Model presents major difficulties, portions of the model can be implemented in any primary care practice—whether a small private office or a large delivery system [33]. A long journey begins with a single step. Ultimately, implementation of the Chronic Care Model signifies a major redesign of medical practice. In the meantime, the model can guide primary care practices to take the first steps toward improving chronic illness care.

Two central messages of the Chronic Care Model are planned care and population-based care. Population-based care requires a registry, but once the registry is in place, physicians are not needed to use the registry for managing their patient panels. Billing personnel, receptionists, medical assistants, or volunteer students—trained to do population management—can sort the registry or registries (a registry might contain one chronic condition like diabetes or multiple conditions) to risk-stratify patients who need more intensive care and make proper appointments for them, to order laboratory tests for patients overdue for such studies, and to arrange care for patients who have not been in contact for a year. Nonphysician personnel can also utilize registries to create and act on reminder prompts and to produce performance feedback reports for the entire practice and for individual clinicians or teams.

Instituting planned care is more of a challenge because it fundamentally changes the entire conception of primary care. Planned care sets aside protected time with care managers to address patient education, self-management support, and clinical management of chronic illness. Until patients become good self-managers (see Chapter 5), planned care requires lengthy and regular encounters. Studies show that a physician with a 2500-patient panel would spend 18 hours per day providing evidence-based chronic and preventive care [11, 12]—an impossible task. Because time is the central bottleneck for physicians, most planned care should be done by nonphysician caregivers, as individual or group visits, by phone, e-mail, or Internet. Planned care requires that physician-centered care be replaced by team-centered care (see Chapter 9).

Who should be the care managers providing planned care? In large organizations, nurses, pharmacists, nutritionists, health educators, and (for asthma and chronic obstructive pulmonary disease) respiratory therapists can be provided with protocols and trained to do planned visits. In small practices, planned care could be provided by nurse practitioners or physician assistants; in the absence of these professionals, some elements of planned care—particularly self-management support—can be offered by medical assistants if time is carved out. Alternatively, small practices could make agreements with hospitals, independent practice associations, or community organizations with personnel who could be trained to provide planned visits. In this era of quality reporting and pay-for-performance, planned visits are an effective way to improve clinical outcomes.

The content of planned visits depends on the training and legal restrictions of the care manager. Often, registered nurses and pharmacists can initiate and titrate medications under physician-approved protocols. In the case of less-trained caregivers, planned visits focus on patient education, self-management support, and—working with the registry—arranging all indicated laboratory studies and other referrals; these planned visits require brief clinician involvement for medication management.

Should planned visits be disease specific? On the one hand, different conditions require care managers to provide different information and skills training to patients. On the other hand, most patients with a chronic condition have more than one condition [34, 35]. In the case of the Chronic Disease Self-Management Program (see Chapter 5), patients with a variety of chronic conditions participate in the same planned care groups. For small practices, medical assistants could be trained to provide self-management support and work the registry for a variety of chronic conditions.

In large practices, or for small practices using care managers at a hospital or other institution, planned visits for disease clusters are a compromise between overly general and excessively specific planned care. A robust, planned visit program would involve at least four categories of care managers: (1) cardiovascular risk reduction and diabetes—including the management of hyperlipidemia, hypertension, obesity, metabolic syndrome, diabetes, smoking cessation, stable coronary heart disease, and CHF (care managers could be nurses, pharmacists, nutritionists, or health educators, some of whom might be certified diabetes educators); (2) asthma and chronic obstructive pulmonary disease (care managers being nurses, pharmacists, or respiratory therapists); (3) arthritis and musculoskeletal conditions (physical or occupational therapists are the ideal care managers); and (4) HIV/AIDS (human immunodeficiency virus/acquired immunodeficiency syndrome), using a multidisciplinary team of clinician, pharmacist, health educator, and social worker. Care managers for all these disease-cluster-specific teams would be trained in the management of depression and pain management, frequent comorbidities to all chronic conditions.

Do all patients with chronic conditions need planned care, and do they need it temporarily or permanently? Often, planned visits are provided to patients exhibiting poor control of their chronic condition, but when the patient has improved, the planned visits stop. It is the impression of a number of clinicians that control (e.g., Hb A1c, LDL cholesterol, and blood pressure) falters when patients return to undifferentiated primary care. The evidence discussed in Chapter 5 confirms these impressions: regular and sustained follow-up is needed to prevent planned-care-associated improvements in clinical outcomes from sliding backwards when planned care, including self-management support, is withdrawn. While some patients highly successful in self-managing their chronic condition can go on autopilot, requiring little assistance from the health care system, most appear to require sustained interactions with planned care. It is highly likely that all patients with chronic conditions should be in contact (face-to-face, phone, or electronic) with planned care on a permanent basis.

In a primary care practice with a planned care team, who is ultimately responsible for the management of chronic conditions? It can be argued that the institutionalization of the Chronic Care Model requires a fundamental redivision of labor within primary care. Physicians do acute care, complex chronic care, and acute exacerbations of chronic care. Nonphysicians do routine chronic care, patient education and skills training, and preventive care. That means separating the acute and complex functions from the routine chronic and preventive work. Ideally, these functions would be housed in the same facility, but in the case of small practices, they may be physically separated. In such a team-based system, patients would be triaged to the physician for acute and complex problems and to the proper care manager for routine chronic and preventive care. Either a care manager or another member of the team would handle registries, reminder prompts, laboratory requisitions, and some patient education functions. Nonphysician team members would function using physician-approved standing orders or protocols. Each activity and each team member would have a distinct, focused, achievable, and measurable mission, replacing the current primary care enterprise with its often vague, general, and unattainable goals.

Such a team-based system might relieve the physician of responsibility for routine, chronic, and preventive care. That responsibility would devolve to the care managers and those caregivers performing the population-based tasks. The physician would approve all protocols, provide training, and oversight and mentor other team members. Many physicians are reluctant to cede responsibility for routine chronic and preventive care to other caregivers; the alternative, however, is for physicians to retain control of an impossible array of tasks, a situation that compromises clinical outcomes.

Will patients allow their routine chronic and preventive care to be provided by nonphysician caregivers? Many practices have found that patients are less likely to attend planned care visits than acute visits. However, if planned care is performed in a relaxed and patient-centered manner, patients begin to accept nonphysician care managers as equals or superior to physicians in chronic care. It is likely that patients who have never experienced team-based care would say no. But patients whose physicians explain to them how the team works, who is responsible for what, and that the physician oversights the other team members, usually accept and then embrace the team system with care managers. Generally, the experiences of primary care practices that have introduced team-based care find that patients want to have their own physician, but understand that the physician will not be present at every encounter.

CONCLUSION

The Chronic Care Model involves a fundamental reorganization of primary care, in which routine chronic and preventive care tasks are separated from acute care and complex chronic care, with nonphysician caregivers assuming the functions of population-based care and planned care. A large body of evidence finds that planned care is associated with improved clinical outcomes for a variety of chronic conditions. The ultimate goal of the Chronic Care Model—to assist patients to become informed and activated self-managers of their chronic conditions—is further discussed in Chapter 5.

REFERENCES

1. Hoffman C, Rice D, Sung HY: Persons with chronic conditions: their prevalence and costs. JAMA. 1996;276:1473–1479.
2. Wagner EH: Meeting the needs of chronically ill people. BMJ. 2001;323:945–946.

3. Chobanian AV, Bakris GL, Black HR, et al: The seventh report of the Joint National Committee on Prevention, Detection, Evaluation, and Treatment of High Blood Pressure. JAMA. 2003;289:2560–2572.

4. Saydah SH, Fradkin J, Cowie CC: Poor control of risk factors for vascular disease among adults with previously diagnosed diabetes. JAMA. 2004;291:335–342.

5. Perez-Stable EJ, Fuentes-Afflick E: Role of clinicians in cigarette smoking prevention. West J Med. 1998;169:23–29.

6. Ni H, Nauman DJ, Hershberger RE: Managed care and outcomes of hospitalization among elderly patients with congestive heart failure. Arch Intern Med. 1998;158:1231–1236.

7. Samsa GP, Matchar DB, Goldstein LB, et al: Quality of anticoagulation management among patients with atrial fibrillation. Arch Intern Med. 2000;160:967–973.

8. Legorreta AP, Liu X, Zaher CA, et al: Variation in managing asthma: experience at the medical group level in California. Am J Manag Care. 2000;6:445–453.

9. Young AS, Klap R, Sherbourne CD, et al: The quality of care for depressive and anxiety disorders in the United States. Arch Gen Psychiatry. 2001;58:55–61.

10. Wagner EH, Austin BT, Von Korff M: Organizing care for patients with chronic illness. Milbank Q. 1996;74:511–544.

11. Ostbye T, Yarnall KSH, Krause DM, et al: Is there time for management of patients with chronic disease in primary care? Ann Fam Med. 2005;3:209–214.

12. Yarnall KS, Pollak KI, Ostbye T, et al: Primary care: is there enough time for prevention? Am J Public Health. 2003;93:635–641.

13. Wagner EH, Austin BT, Davis C, et al: Improving chronic illness care: translating evidence into action. Health Aff. 2001;20(6):64–78.

14. Bodenheimer T, Wagner EH, Grumbach K: Improving primary care for patients with chronic illness. JAMA. 2002;288:1775–1779.

15. Bodenheimer T, Wagner EH, Grumbach K: Improving primary care for patients with chronic illness: the chronic care model, Part 2. JAMA. 2002;288:1909–1914.

16. Schmittdiel J, Bodenheimer T, Solomon NA, et al: The prevalence and use of chronic disease registries in physician organizations. J Gen Intern Med. 2005;20:855–858.

17. Nuovo J (ed.). *Chronic Disease Management*. New York, Springer, 2006.

18. Glasgow RE, Orleans CT, Wagner EH: Does the chronic care model serve also as a template for improving prevention? Milbank Q. 2001;79:579–612.

19. Sperl-Hillen JM, O'Connor PJ: Factors driving diabetes care improvement in a large medical group: ten years of progress. Am J Managed Care. 2005;11:S177–S185.

20. Wagner EH: Quality improvement in chronic illness care: a collaborative approach. Jt Comm J Qual Improv. 2001;27:63–80.
21. Fireman B, Bartlett J, Selby J: Can disease management reduce health care costs by improving quality? Health Aff. 2004;23(6):63–75.
22. Gwadry-Sridhar FH, Flintoft V, Lee DS, et al: A systematic review and meta-analysis of studies comparing readmission rates and mortality rates in patients with heart failure. Arch Intern Med. 2004;164:2315–2320.
23. Holland R. Battersby J, Harvey I, et al: Systematic review of multidisciplinary interventions in heart failure. Heart 2005;91:899–906.
24. McAlister FA, Lawson FME, Teo KK, et al: A systematic review of randomized trials of disease management programs in heart failure. Am J Med. 2001;110;378–384.
25. Wagner EH: Deconstructing heart failure disease management. Ann Intern Med. 2004;131:644–646.
26. Tinkelman D, Wilson S: Asthma disease management: regression to the mean or better? Am J Manag Care. 2004;10:948–954.
27. McAlister FA, Lawson FME, Teo KK, et al: Randomized trials of secondary prevention programmes in coronary heart disease: a systematic review. BMJ. 2001;323:957–962.
28. Raftery JP, Yao GL, Murchie P, et al: Cost effectiveness of nurse led secondary prevention clinics for coronary heart disease in primary care. BMJ. 2005;330:707–710.
29. Villagra VG, Ahmed T: Effectiveness of a disease management program for patients with diabetes. Health Aff. 2004;23(4):255–266.
30. Congressional Budget Office: An Analysis of the Literature on Disease Management Programs, October 13, 2004. (*www.cbo.gov*)
31. Crosson FJ, Madvig P: Does population management of chronic disease lead to lower costs of care? Health Aff. 2004;23(6):76–78.
32. Krause DS: Economic effectiveness of disease management programs. Dis Manag. 2005;8:114–134.
33. Mohler PJ, Mohler NB. Improving chronic illness care: lessons learned in a private practice. Fam Pract Manag. 2005;12(10):50–56.
34. Starfield B, Lemke KW, Bernhardt T, et al: Comorbidity: implications for the importance of primary care in 'case' management. Ann Fam Med. 2003;1:8–14.
35. Grumbach K: Chronic illness, comorbidities, and the need for medical generalists. Ann Fam Med. 2003;1:4–7.

CHAPTER FIVE

Self-Management Support for People with Chronic Illness

Self-management is what people do every day: decide what to eat, whether to exercise, if and when they will monitor their health, or take medications [1]. Self-management refers to the day-to-day tasks an individual does or does not undertake to prevent, control, or reduce the impact of a chronic condition. Everyone self-manages; the question is whether people make decisions that improve their health-related behaviors and clinical outcomes. People who are motivated to make daily decisions and choose actions favoring healthy behaviors are sometimes called *good self-managers*.

Self-management support is what health caregivers do to assist and encourage patients to become good self-managers [1]. The simplest definition of self-management support is "including patients in their own care" [2]. The Institute of Medicine's definition is "the systematic provision of education and supportive interventions to increase patients' skills and confidence in managing their health problems, including regular assessment of progress and problems, goal setting, and problem-solving support" [3].

To become a good self-manager, people need to have (1) an understanding of the chronic condition they wish to prevent or improve, and

(2) self-motivation to choose and engage in healthy behaviors. Good self-managers are informed and activated individuals. For healthy people, good self-management involves making illness-preventing choices regarding diet, exercise, use of addictive substances, and participation in clinical preventive activities such as Pap smears, mammograms, and blood pressure and cholesterol screening. For people with chronic illness, good self-managers make the same behavioral choices and also regularly self-monitor and self-adjust their chronic condition, and take appropriate medications. In addition, good self-managers have learned to cope with the emotional toll of chronic illness and use problem-solving skills to overcome the day-to-day stresses that accompany a chronic condition.

Good self-managers possess considerable knowledge, multiple skills including problem solving, and an inner motivation to put their knowledge and skills to work on a daily basis. Self-management support involves two interrelated activities [4]:

- Providing information and skills training about the chronic condition that a person has or about illness prevention (assisting people to become informed)

- Helping people to become the major participant in preventing, managing, and coping with a chronic condition(s) (encouraging people to become activated)

The purpose of self-management support is to assist and encourage people to become informed and activated, both for preventive and chronic care. The distinction between preventive and chronic care is a fuzzy one—after all, chronic care management largely consists of secondary prevention.

Some people become good self-managers without help from the health care system. Other people never become motivated to make healthy choices no matter how much assistance they receive. The majority of people become better self-managers if they receive high-quality self-management support on a regular and permanent basis.

TRADITIONAL VERSUS COLLABORATIVE RELATIONSHIPS

Louise is a health educator at a community health center. She received her health education training 40 years ago and is near retirement. She teaches people with diabetes the 26 knowledge and skills domains recommended by the American Diabetes Association. She offers the domains in logical order and tests her patients on the knowledge they have gained. She was taught that when patients understand their diabetes, they gain better control of their condition. When her patients fail to improve their Hb A1c levels she feels that they are not studying hard enough. She mentors a young health education student, but is dissatisfied because the student won't teach the 26 domains in a logical order.

Cindy just received her masters in health education and began to work at a public hospital family health center. A product of new collaborative theories, she starts her individual or group diabetes sessions by asking, "Is there anything you would like to know about your diabetes?" She tries to cover all areas of knowledge, but the knowledge is provided as answers to patients' curiosity rather than as a planned syllabus.

Patients do not bring a list of home-monitored glucose values for Cindy to interpret; rather, they are trained to understand the significance of high or low sugar and its relation to food and exercise, and are taught to self-adjust their diet, exercise, or medications depending on the glucose levels at different times of the day. For Cindy, self-monitoring means that patients make measurements and react to those measurements themselves, rather than depending on the health care system to make the adjustments.

Cindy also spends time encouraging patients to set goals, such as losing 5 pounds, or reducing the LDL-C by 30 points. She makes action plans with patients—concrete activities that help in attaining the patients' goals. She finds that goal setting and action planning increase people's self-confidence that they can take control of their diabetes.

Many people mistakenly think that self-management support is the same as patient education. In fact, self-management support involves a fundamental paradigm shift in the patient-caregiver relationship [5]. In the traditional paradigm, caregivers, particularly physicians, tell patients what to do to improve their health. The new paradigm builds a partnership between caregiver and patient, with shared responsibility for making and carrying out health-related decisions. In contrast to Louise whose activities focus on imparting knowledge, caregivers like Cindy provide knowledge, skills including problem-solving skills, tools, and encouragement. One aspect of the paradigm shift involves moving away from the didactic model of patient education utilized by Louise toward Cindy's method of providing information that the patient is interested in learning.

Some characteristics of the paradigm shift from traditional to collaborative interactions are listed in Table 5–1.

TABLE 5–1
The Paradigm Shift

Traditional interactions
- Information is provided based on the caregiver's agenda
- Belief that knowledge is sufficient to create behavior change
- Goal is compliance with the caregiver's advice
- Decisions are made by the caregiver

Collaborative interactions
- Information and skills training are provided based on the patient's agenda
- Belief that self-efficacy (confidence in ability to change) creates behavior change
- Goal is increased self-efficacy, not compliance with caregiver's advice
- Decisions are made as a patient-caregiver partnership

Self-efficacy, a key concept in self-management, refers to a person's confidence that he or she can carry out a behavior necessary to reach a desired goal. In the words of Kate Lorig, a pioneer in the field of chronic disease self-management, "If people think they can do something, they probably can. If people don't think they can do something, they probably can't do it." A number of studies demonstrate that self-efficacy is associated with healthier behaviors [6].

Is self-management support pertinent to all patients or are some patients by nature passive, poorly motivated, and unable to self-manage? Some patients are by nature passive, but caregivers should use self-management tools (described below) to try to activate and inform them. If a patient chooses not to participate in health-related decisions, preferring that the clinician advise him or her what to do, the clinician has no choice but to make decisions on behalf of the patient but should check each time to ensure that the patient agrees.

IMPLEMENTING SELF-MANAGEMENT SUPPORT IN CLINICAL PRACTICE: THE 5 A'S

In 1989, the National Cancer Institute developed a multicomponent program to guide physicians in assisting patients to stop smoking. This framework, which has changed over time, is now known as the 5 A's:

assess (ask), advise, agree, assist, and arrange. The U.S. Preventive Services Task Force has chosen the 5 A's to serve as a unifying construct in describing counseling interventions for a variety of health-related behaviors [7]. While many self-management support activities partake of several of the 5 A's, the construct is useful to teach caregivers practical tools and strategies for providing self-management support.

Assess (Ask)

Assessment involves two areas: medical and motivational. The medical component of assessment involves asking whether the patient has one or more chronic conditions, the severity of the condition(s), how well or poorly the patient is self-managing the condition(s), and what the patient knows and wants to know about the condition(s). For patients without a chronic condition, assessment involves determination of the patient's health-related behaviors and the level of risk that the patient will develop a chronic condition.

The motivational component of assessment involves asking whether patients have a desire to improve health-related behaviors (including management of chronic illness) and an understanding of the barriers preventing patients from becoming activated self-managers. The assessment of motivation has become known as determining a patient's *readiness to change*.

There are two related but distinct ways to think about readiness to change. One, the *stages of change* construct, is widely taught in health professional schools; its simplicity has made it a popular, but potentially hazardous, formula for assessing motivation. The stages of change model classifies individuals into one of the following groups based on their readiness to change: precontemplation (not intending to make a behavior change during the following 6 months), contemplation (thinking about behavior change), preparation (intending to take action within a month), action (making a specific change), and maintenance (prevention of relapse, with the behavior change persisting for 6 months to 5 years) [8].

The other readiness to change formulation—offered by theorists of Motivational Interviewing—does not pigeonhole patients into specific stages. Motivational Interviewing (MI) is a counseling approach that fits within the collaborative paradigm of self-management support [9]. In the MI model, readiness = importance × confidence. For example, people who do not think physical activity is important are unlikely to begin such activity. People who view physical activity as important but lack confidence (self-efficacy) in their ability to succeed are similarly unlikely to initiate the change. Unlike the *precontemplation* stage of change, which lumps all nonready people together, the MI concept perceives that the interventions needed to encourage change when low importance is the barrier, are different than those needed when low confidence is the issue. For low importance, patient education is needed, whereas for low confidence, the indicated tools are goal setting, action planning, and problem solving (described below) [10]. An example of motivational assessment is provided in Appendix L.

The stages-of-change concept may be useful in assessing motivation for stopping a specific addiction (smoking or alcohol), but does not apply to self-management behaviors concerned with prevention and chronic care [11]. A review of 87 studies based on stages of change found no empirical evidence to suggest that the stages are discrete [12]. A separate systematic review of 37 trials found little evidence that stage-based approaches to behavior change are more effective than non-staged-based strategies [13]. Patients may be involved in more than one stage at the same time, and evidence cannot confirm that behavior change occurs in distinct stages [11].

Advise

The second *A*—advise—refers to information giving: patient education and skills training. It is also connected with the *importance* component of the motivation assessment. Information helps patients appreciate the importance of making a behavior change—whether diet, exercise, self-monitoring of blood sugars, or taking medications regularly—and may increase motivation.

It is well-known that patients with chronic conditions do not receive enough information. In a 1994 study, 76% of patients with type 2 diabetes received limited or no diabetes education [14]. As many as 50% of patients leave an office visit not understanding what they were told by the physician [15]. Minority patients receive less information about tests, procedures, treatments, and prognosis than White patients [16].

Other times, patients are bombarded with too much information. For example, the American Diabetes Association (ADA) Web site lists 26 domains of knowledge and skill building for patients with diabetes. Walking through this curriculum step-by-step may impart more confusion than useful knowledge. Adult learning takes place chiefly through *self-directed learning*, in which the material to be learned is chosen by the learner, and does not follow a step-by-step or linear format.

Ask-Tell-Ask: Miller and Rollnick, in their book *Motivational Interviewing* [17], describe a technique that provides information to patients (addressing the lack-of-information problem) in a manner directed by the patient (solving the excess-of-information problem). This technique can be called *ask-tell-ask*. For example, a caregiver asks a patient newly diagnosed with diabetes, "What do you know about diabetes?" and "What would you like to know about diabetes?" After receiving an answer, the caregiver then tells the patient the information, and thereafter, asks if the patient understood and what additional information is desired. Over time, many of ADA's 26 domains may be covered, but via a patient-directed agenda. An ask-tell-ask discussion is demonstrated in Appendix L.

Closing-the-Loop: Related to ask-tell-ask is an important process called *closing-the-loop* or *teach-back*. According to Schillinger and colleagues, in only 12% of discussions providing new advice (a lifestyle change recommendation or new medication) did physicians ask patients with diabetes to restate the physician's instructions—indicating that they understood what the physician said. This technique of assessing a patient's understanding is called closing-the-loop. When patients were asked to restate the information given by the physician, they responded incorrectly 47% of the time. In the study, patients given the opportunity to close the loop had average Hb A1c levels lower than patients who were not given the opportunity to restate what they were told. Closing-the-loop, a simple technique of assessing patients' understanding, can improve patient comprehension and diabetes outcomes [18]. A closing-the-loop discussion example is provided in Appendix L.

Skills Training: Teaching self-monitoring skills is an important part of information giving. However, skills training which does not teach the patient to interpret the monitored measures is inadequate. Many people with diabetes learn to check their sugars, but do not know the meaning of the numbers on the glucometer. True self-monitoring training provides patients with expertise in self-regulation; for example, if sugars are too high in the morning and too low in the late afternoon, the patient knows to take more medication at night and less in the morning, and to adjust eating or exercise routines. Good self-managers rarely rely on the health care system to make these adjustments.

Information is Not Enough: In the past, many people believed that providing information to patients would, by itself, improve health-related behaviors. This belief has been conclusively refuted.

A comprehensive review of diabetes patient education found that in 33 out of 46 studies, education improved patients' knowledge about their condition, but in only 18 of 54 studies did patient education improve the control of blood sugar levels [19]. An analysis of 59 trials of hypertension management found that patient education alone does not improve blood pressures [20]. A review of 12 asthma studies concluded that patient education alone did not improve asthma-related symptoms and did not reduce the frequency of asthma-related visits to the emergency department [21]. Similar findings have been published for arthritis [22]. Nor did education increase the extent to which patients actually took prescribed medications [23].

Information is necessary but not sufficient to encourage healthier behaviors and improved clinical outcomes; the other critical elements are included in the next 3 A's: agree, assist, and arrange.

Agree

In the traditional paradigm, the physician advises the patient to make lifestyle changes: "You need to stop smoking." "If you want to get your diabetes under control, you've got to exercise 30 minutes a day."

In the collaborative paradigm, improving health-related behaviors is a decision the patient needs to make. In Kate Lorig's experience, "If people don't want to do something, they won't do it." Under the collaborative paradigm, an agenda for the visit is negotiated between the patient and caregiver, but the patient has the last word. If the caregiver wishes to discuss an issue with the patient, the patient's permission for that discussion should be sought.

Let us assume that in the agenda-setting process, the patient agrees to discuss making a health-related behavior change. A collaborative way to initiate a behavior change discussion is to ask the question used by Kate Lorig in self-management classes: "Is there anything you would like to do this week to improve your health?" The Kate Lorig question allows patients to choose which behavior they are motivated to change, and forms the basis for agreement on a self-management goal (Table 5–2).

Cindy asks Mr. Jorge Fuentes "Is there anything you would like to do this week to improve your health?" Mr. Fuentes: "I know I'm eating too

TABLE 5–2
The Kate Lorig question
Is there anything you would like to do this week to improve your health?

much but I can't change that right now. Maybe I could get off my butt and do more exercise." Mr. Fuentes has made a general exercise goal, but it is neither concrete nor measurable. When Cindy asks if he would like to make a specific action plan to achieve the goal, Mr. Fuentes promises to walk 3 miles each day. Cindy asks how sure he is that he can go from no exercise to 3 miles each day. On a confidence scale of 0 to 10, Mr. Fuentes says it's a 2. Understanding that success is more important than the amount of exercise, Cindy suggests making an action plan with a high chance of success. After a discussion, they agree that Mr. Fuentes will walk for 15 minutes after lunch each Monday, Wednesday, and Friday. Cindy promises to call him the following week to see how he is doing with his action plan.

Goal setting involves patients and caregivers agreeing on a general self-management goal, for example, reducing the Hb A1c from 9 to 7 or losing 10 pounds. Action plans (Figure 5–1) are concrete and specific activities a patient agrees to do to help reach the goal; for example, walking around the block twice on Mondays, Wednesdays, and Saturdays before lunch, or reducing consumption of cookies from three to one per day [5]. With nonspecific goals, for example, to exercise or lose weight, patients cannot evaluate their success and often experience failure. To enhance the likelihood that patients will succeed, clinicians ask patients to estimate, on a 0–10 scale, how confident they are that they can carry out the action plan. Action plans can be downsized such that patient have a confidence level of at least 7/10 that they can succeed (Figure 5–1). A goal-setting dialogue is furnished in Appendix L. Action plan forms in English, Spanish, and Chinese are available at: (*www.familymedicine.medschool.ucsf.edu/research/research_programs/actionPlan.aspx*)

Evidence is emerging that goal setting and action planning are effective across the socioeconomic spectrum. In one study, low-income patients receiving care in safety net clinics were able to initiate behavior changes based on action plans as often as higher-income patients in private practices [24].

The theoretical basis for goal setting and action planning is the concept of self-efficacy—a person's confidence that he or she can carry out a

DATE: _____

MY ACTION PLAN

I _____and _____
            (name)   (name of clinician)

have agreed that to improve my health I will:

1. Choose one of the activities below:	2. Choose your confidence level:
_____Work on something that's bothering me: _____	This is how sure I am that I will be able to do my action plan:
_____Stay more physically active!	10 VERY SURE
	5 SOMEWHAT SURE
_____Take my medications.	0 NOT SURE AT ALL
	3. Complete this box for the chosen activity:
	What:_____ _____
_____Improve my food choices.	How much:_____
	When:_____ _____
_____Reduce my stress.	How often:_____
_____Cut down on smoking.	_____ (Signature)
	_____ (Signature of clinician)

FIGURE 5–1. Action plan form.

behavior necessary to reach a desired goal. Studies from non-health-related industries conclude that a specific goal leads to higher performance than no goal or a vague goal such as "do your best." In addition, proximal goals (short-term and specific) are associated with better performance than distal (long-term and general) goals. Setting proximal subgoals (action plans) makes the reward of success come sooner and increases self-efficacy. Increased self-efficacy results in people setting and achieving higher goals, while reduced self-efficacy—from failing to achieve a goal—may lead to goal abandonment [25]. In health-related behavior change, self-efficacy is also associated with healthier behaviors [6].

Several reviews suggest that goal setting and action planning are associated with improved health-related behaviors, though the evidence is not conclusive [26]. A review of 92 studies of diet behaviors found that goal setting or action planning were associated with the eating of less fat and more fruits and vegetables [27]. Another review of 28 studies on diet and physical activity found that 32% of the studies supported the use of goal setting or action planning for adults; the literature for adolescents and children is limited [28]. The Agency for Healthcare Research and Quality included goal setting in a list of counseling components to improve diet [29]. The American Diabetes Association, the American Association of Diabetes Educators, and the American Heart Association recommend goal setting as one component of cardiovascular disease risk reduction. It is safe to say that goal setting and action planning, in conjunction with other self-management support components, appear to improve health-related behaviors.

To summarize, the third A—agree—involves the caregiver and patient agreeing on an agenda for the visit, and—if the patient is in agreement—collaboratively setting a goal and making an action plan.

Assist

Assist (Table 5–3) refers to caregiver activities that "address barriers to change, increase the patient's motivation and self-help skills, and/or help the patient secure the needed supports for successful behavior change" [7].

Assistance can be provided prior to the patient agreeing on a self-management goal or after the patient sets a goal and makes an action plan.

Assistance Prior to Setting a Goal: *Cindy was delighted that Mr. Fuentes was succeeding at his exercise action plan. She reassessed his motivation to improve his diet, and utilized an MI technique to explore Mr. Fuentes' ambivalence. Mr. Fuentes agreed that it was important to improve his diet because he was an amateur photographer and he was afraid his diabetes would cause him to go blind. Cindy assessed that statement as change*

TABLE 5–3
Assisting Patients to Develop Self-Management Skills

Teaching of self-monitoring skills

Motivational interviewing to encourage patient involvement and activation

Reviewing goals and action plans to identify problems

Teaching problem-solving skills

Offering coping skills (*Living a healthy life with a chronic condition*), including

- Dealing with pain, shortness of breath, other symptoms
- Adjusting to restricted functioning
- Overcoming depression, anxiety, hopelessness

---

talk—that Mr. Fuentes was trying to convince himself to do something about the diet. But Mr. Fuentes' confidence level that he could succeed was only 3 on a scale of 0-10. Cindy asked "What would raise your confidence level from a 3 to a 7?" Mr. Fuentes said he would be more confident if he didn't get pizza for lunch with his friend at work. Cindy suggested making an action plan regarding those lunches. After a discussion, they agreed that tomorrow at lunch he would talk to his friend, who had high cholesterol, to consider bringing healthy lunches to work and eating together at the park four blocks away. Cindy promised to call the following evening to see what happened.

In helping patients address barriers to change, caregivers trained in MI do not convince people to adopt healthy behaviors. MI assumes that most people are ambivalent about whether or not to change behaviors and tries to bring the ambivalence out in the open. Ideally, it is the patient, not the caregiver, who presents the argument for change. MI counseling encourages *change talk*—patients making arguments about why behavior change would be a good idea. Mr. Fuentes' concern about his eyes prompted him to make change talk about the need to improve his diet.

Reviews of Motivational Interviewing find some evidence of success for drug and alcohol addiction, weight reduction, and blood pressure control; the effectiveness of MI in smoking cessation, enhancing physical activity, and managing chronic illness is inconclusive [1, 10]. Motivational Interviewing may be particularly effective with individuals assessed to have low motivation to change [30]. Because MI counselors vary greatly in competence, its effectiveness may be more related to the skill of the counselor than to any other factor [9].

Assistance after Setting a Goal: When Cindy called Mr. Fuentes the next evening, she found him discouraged. His friend agreed that pizza was unhealthy, but described a family situation that would make it impossible to prepare lunch at home. Cindy helped Mr. Fuentes to solve the problem, asking *"Do you have any ideas on what you might do instead of eating pizza that would not require your friend to bring lunch from home?"* Mr. Fuentes suggested that he and his friend might eat at the deli five blocks from work where soup, salad, and low-fat sandwiches were served. The following day, his friend agreed to that plan, and a new action plan was made to eat every weekday at the deli instead of the pizza place.

Frequently, action plans run into unforeseen obstacles. Problem solving is a skill that allows people to overcome the obstacles (see Appendix L for a simple problem-solving method). A basic trio of self-management skills includes goal setting, action planning, and problem solving.

The Evidence for Programs that Assist Patients: Many studies have explored the use of a variety of programs to assist people in self-managing several chronic conditions. A review of eight studies found that diabetes empowerment training—teaching goal setting, action plans, problem solving, and coping skills—was associated with improved Hb A1c levels compared with controls [31, 32]. Fifteen studies featuring nurses or pharmacists providing patient-centered counseling for patients with hypertension improved blood pressures compared with patients receiving usual care [33].

Assisting patients with asthma is an interesting story. The 1997 NIH Expert Panel's Guidelines for the Diagnosis and Management of Asthma (updated in 2002) states, "Patients should be given a written action plan and be instructed how to use it" [34]. Many physicians use asthma action plans in managing their patients with asthma.

Asthma action plans are not the same as behavior-change action plans. They are a true self-monitoring and self-care tool. Patients are given a red, yellow, and green form, the asthma action plan, which lists the symptoms (or the readings from a peak flow meter) related to good asthma control (green), worsening asthma (yellow), and serious exacerbation (red). Each day patients are encouraged to self-monitor whether they are in the green, yellow, or red zone. If they are in the yellow zone, they increase their medications; in the red danger zone, they increase medications and seek immediate medical assistance. Asthma action plans are analogous to self-monitoring taught to heart failure patients—to weigh themselves daily and increase their diuretics if the weight increases above a certain level—or to patients with diabetes—to increase their medications and exercise and to reduce food intake if their blood sugars rise above a certain level. Patients' ability to conduct this kind of self-monitoring and adjustment is the essence of a good self-manager, who is no longer so dependent on the health care system.

In spite of widespread acceptance of asthma action plans, the evidence supporting their use is controversial. Two separate reviews, one from the highly respected Cochrane Collaboration, concluded that asthma action plans do not reduce asthma hospitalizations, emergency department, or urgent physician visits, or—for children—days lost from school [35, 36]. Another Cochrane review found the opposite, stating that patient self-adjustment of medications using asthma action plans is as good as physician's adjustment of medications [37]. If patients are trained, they do it as well as doctors. This controversy is revisited later in this chapter.

The management of chronic atrial fibrillation using the anticoagulant warfarin provides strong evidence for the effectiveness of patient self-adjustment of medications. Warfarin treatment requires that a blood test, the INR (International Normalized Ratio—blood clotting measure), be maintained in a narrow range; too much warfarin resulting in a high INR can lead to hemorrhage while insufficient warfarin causing a low INR increases the risk of a stroke. A 2004 literature review concluded that patients who self-monitor and self-adjust their warfarin dose at home have INR levels in the target range more frequently than patients whose physicians adjust doses. Those patients who choose self-regulation perform better than their physicians [38, 39].

Arthritis was the condition that jump-started the entire field of chronic disease self-management. Kate Lorig and Halsted Holman at Stanford University created the Arthritis Self-Management Program (ASMP), also known as the Arthritis Self-Help Program or Challenging Arthritis. Arthritis patients attending a six-session self-management class were compared with a usual-care control group. The class offered problem-solving skills, action plans, and efforts to improve self-efficacy. Four years after patients participated in the course, they reported a mean reduction in pain symptoms of 20%; the comparison group did not demonstrate this improvement. Improvement was associated with growth of self-efficacy by improving patient confidence in being able to cope with their chronic condition [40]. The ASMP has been replicated at other institutions, and a total of eight studies have been published on this self-management program, all of them showing improved outcomes compared with controls [5].

Kate Lorig expanded the ASMP into the Chronic Disease Self-Management Program (CDSMP). Patients with a variety of chronic conditions met together in seven weekly classes teaching goal setting, action plans, problem solving, and coping skills [41]. Six months after attending the classes, participants improved control of their symptoms and demonstrated a reduction in limitation of activity compared with controls [42]. After 2 years, course participants maintained improved scores on scales measuring self-efficacy and health distress [43].

In summary, a variety of self-management support programs have been shown to improve outcomes for several common chronic conditions. It should be clear that the A's in the 5 A's are closely intertwined and that the more A's the better.

Arrange

Self-management support is not a short-term activity; it should involve regular, sustained follow-up. *Arrange* refers to follow-up, whether the follow-up is conducted by the caregivers who initiated the self-management support or through referral to programs in other health care or community settings. Follow-up can be arranged—depending on what is available and on patient preference—through regular visits, telephone, e-mail, specialized counseling services, or community-based facilities for healthy eating, exercise, or treatment of addictions. Follow-up may be done through programs that bring patients together into groups or through buddy systems with patients doing self-management tasks in pairs. These arrangements, which turn patients into caregivers, allow patients to help each other, and reduce the burden on the health care system.

A large body of evidence demonstrates the importance of regular, sustained follow-up. A Cochrane Review found that patients with diabetes who had regular follow-up had better Hb A1c levels than patients without follow-up [44]. In a meta-analysis, Norris and colleagues showed that the benefits of self-management support for patients with diabetes diminish over time, that regular follow-up is needed, and that the total time caregivers spend with patients is closely correlated with improved glycemic control [45]. Clement's review of diabetes self-management emphasizes that follow-up is key to long-term success [14]. The Diabetes Prevention Program, the landmark study showing that lifestyle changes alone reduced the number of people with impaired glucose tolerance who developed frank diabetes by 58%, kept the intervention group faithful to the lifestyle changes by unrelenting follow-up [46]. Similar to the case of diabetes, regular follow-up—as shown by a review of 59 trials—is necessary for the management of hypertension [20].

The discussion of *assist* above left uncertain whether asthma action plans are effective in improving asthma outcomes. It turns out that if the asthma action plans are accompanied by regular follow-up, they are effective, if not, they may not work [37].

Self-management support for patients with congestive heart failure (CHF) places a major effort on follow-up. Three separate reviews of many randomized controlled trials of CHF patients discharged from the hospital found that nurse-led follow-up (in the home, in clinics, or by phone) was associated with large reductions in CHF readmissions, and in some cases reductions in mortality [47–49]. The most effective programs are those that begin immediately after hospital discharge and in which some of the follow-up is face-to-face rather than only by telephone [50].

As with all the evidence concerning the 5 A's, studies supporting the necessity of follow-up include other components of self-management support. Follow-up itself involves assessment, advice, agreement, and assistance.

CONCLUSION

Self-management support involves a variety of activities through which caregivers help and encourage patients to become better self-managers. A strong body of evidence shows that self-management support—using a mixture of components—is effective in improving clinical outcomes. Much work, however, is still needed on precisely which activities are the most effective with which patients. From a research perspective, it is difficult to isolate one component of the 5 A's to determine its individual effectiveness. From a caregiving perspective, self-management support needs to include all or most of the 5 A's. Certain things are clear: information alone does not improve clinical outcomes; other components of the 5 A's that involve patients as partners in a collaborative relationship are needed. The triad of goal setting, action planning, and problem solving, while not rigorously evidence based, appear to be important techniques to improve health-related behaviors and clinical outcomes. Finally, regular and sustained follow-up is essential.

In order to implement and sustain self-management support as an expected feature of primary care practice, major changes are needed. The multi-agenda 15-minute physician visit is entirely inadequate as a platform for providing self-management support [4]. While physicians have an important role in encouraging patients to become better self-managers, other members of the health care team need to implement the 5 A's in their work with patients (see Chapter 9). Self-management support cannot be accomplished without the planned visits discussed in Chapter 4. One primary care model would remove routine chronic care management, including self-management support, from the list of physician responsibilities and place it in the hands of a planned care team.

Who is on the planned care team, and whether the team is within or outside of the primary care setting depends on the setting. In small physician practices, some self-management functions—for example, skills training, action planning, and follow-up—could be delegated to trained medical assistants, if they have time to perform these tasks. But small practices are dependent on outside health care and community resources to conduct self-management support. Larger primary care practices with more nonphysician personnel can establish internal planned care teams with the physician as one team member. Ample training in how to do self-management support is needed to create an effective team, because many components of the 5 A's are not taught in most health science schools [51]. An assessment of how well a primary care practice is providing self-management support is provided in Appendix M.

The need to provide self-management support, both for healthy people needing to prevent disease and for those who have one or more chronic conditions, represents a major challenge to primary care. Current structures cannot do the job.

REFERENCES

1. Bodenheimer T, Macgregor K, Sharifi C: *Helping Patients Manage Their Chronic Conditions.* Oakland, CA, California HealthCare Foundation, June 2005 *(www.chcf.org)*
2. Lorig K, Holman H: *Self-Management Education.* Palo Alto, CA, Stanford Patient Education Research Center, 2000.
3. Institute of Medicine. *Priority Areas for National Action: Transforming Health Care Quality.* Washington, DC, National Academies Press, 2003, p 52.

4. Bodenheimer T: Helping patients improve their health-related behaviors: what system changes do we need? Dis Manag. 2005;8:326–337.
5. Bodenheimer T, Lorig K, Holman H, et al: Patient self-management of chronic disease in primary care. JAMA. 2002;288:2469–2475.
6. Marks R, Allegrante JP, Lorig K: A review and synthesis of research evidence for self-efficacy-enhancing interventions for reducing chronic disability. Health Promot Pract. 2005;6:37–43,148–156.
7. Whitlock EP, Orlean CT, Pender N, et al: Evaluating primary care behavioral counseling interventions. Am J Prev Med. 2002;22:267–284.
8. Prochaska JO, Velicer WF: The transtheoretical model of health behavior change. Am J Health Promot. 1997;12:38–48.
9. Resnicow K, DiIorio C, Soet JE, et al: Motivational Interviewing in health promotion. Health Psychol. 2002;21:444–451.
10. Rollnick S, Mason P, Butler C: *Health Behavior Change: A Guide for Practitioners.* Edinburgh, Churchill Livingstone, 2000.
11. Marshall SJ, Biddle SJ: The transtheoretical model of behavior change: a meta-analysis of applications to physical activity and exercise. Ann Behav Med. 2001;23:229–246.
12. Littell JH, Girvin H: Stages of change: A critique. Behav Modif. 2002;26:223–273.
13. Riemsma RP, Pattenden J, Bridle C, et al: A systematic review of the effectiveness of interventions based on a stages-of-change approach to promote individual behaviour change. Health Technol Assess. 2002;6(24): 1–231.
14. Clement S: Diabetes self-management education. Diabetes Care. 1995;18:1204–1214.
15. Roter DL, Hall JA: Studies of doctor-patient interaction. Annu Rev Public Health. 1989;10:163–180.
16. Stewart AL, Napoles-Springer A, Perez-Stable EJ: Interpersonal processes of care in diverse populations. Milbank Q. 1999;77:305–339, 274.
17. Miller WR, Rollnick S: *Motivational Interviewing.* New York, Guilford Press, 2002.
18. Schillinger D, Piette J, Grumbach K, et al: Closing the loop: physician communication with diabetic patients who have low health literacy. Arch Intern Med. 2003;163:83–90.
19. Norris SL, Engelgau MM, Narayan KMV: Effectiveness of self-management training in type 2 diabetes. Diabetes Care. 2001;24:561–587.
20. Fahey T, Schroeder K, Ebrahim S: Interventions used to improve control of blood pressure in patients with hypertension. Cochrane Database Syst Rev. 2005;(1):CD005182.
21. Gibson PG, Powell H, Coughlan J, et al: Limited (information-only) patient education programs for adults with asthma. Cochrane Database Syst Rev. 2002;(1):CD001005.

22. Riemsma RP, Kirwan J, Rasker J, et al: Patient education for adults with rheumatoid arthritis. The Cochrane Database of Systematic Reviews, 2003;(2):CD003688

23. Haynes RB, McDonald H, Garg AX, et al: Interventions for helping patients to follow prescriptions for medications. Cochrane Database Syst Rev. 2002;(2):CD000011.

24. Handley M, MacGregor K, Schillinger D, et al: Using action plans to help primary care patients adopt healthy behaviors. J Amer Board Family Med. 2006;19:224–231.

25. Locke EA, Latham GP: Building a practically useful theory of goal setting and task motivation. Am Psychol. 2002;57:705–717.

26. Goldstein MG, Whitlock EP, DePue J: Multiple behavioral risk factor interventions in primary care: summary of research evidence. Am J Prev Med. 2004; 27(2 Suppl):61–79.

27. Ammerman AS, Lindquist CH, Lohr KN, et al: The efficacy of behavioral interventions to modify dietary fat and fruit and vegetable intake: a review of the evidence. Prev Med. 2002;35:25–41.

28. Shilts MK, Horowitz M, Townsend MS: Goal setting as a strategy for dietary and physical activity behavior change: a review of the literature. Am J Health Promot. 2004;19:81–93.

29. Pignone MP, Ammerman A, Fernandez L, et al: Counseling to promote a healthy diet in adults: a summary of evidence for the U.S. Preventive Services Task Force. Am J Prev Med. 2003;24:75–92.

30. Butler C, Rollnick S, Cohen D, et al: Motivational consulting versus brief advice for smokers in general practice: a randomized trial. Brit J General Practice. 1999;49:611–616.

31. van Dam HA, van der Horst F, van den Borne B, et al: Provider-patient interaction in diabetes care. Patient Educ Couns. 2003;51:17–28.

32. Anderson RM, Funnell MM, Butler PM, et al: Patient empowerment: results of a randomized controlled trial. Diabetes Care. 1995;18:943–949.

33. Boulware LE, Daumit GL, Frick KD, et al: An evidence-based review of patient-centered behavioral interventions for hypertension. Am J Prev Med. 2001;21:221–232.

34. NIH, NHLBI: Expert Panel Report 2, Guidelines for the Diagnosis and Management of Asthma, 1997. (*www.nhlbi.nih.gov/guidelines/asthma/asthupdt.htm*)

35. Toelle BG, Ram FSF: Written individualized management plans for asthma in children and adults. Cochrane Database Syst Rev. 2004;(1):-CD002171.

36. Lefevre F, Piper M, Weiss K, et al: Do written asthma action plans improve patient outcomes in asthma? J Fam Pract. 2002;51:842–848.

37. Powell H, Gibson PG: Options for self-management education for adults with asthma. Cochrane Database Syst Rev. 2003;(1):CD004107

38. Yang DT, Robetorye RS, Rodgers GM: Home prothrombin time monitoring: a literature analysis. Am J Hematol. 2004;77:177–186.
39. Murray E, Fitzmaurice D, McCahon D, et al: Training for patients in a randomized controlled trial of self-management of warfarin treatment. BMJ. 2004;328:437–438.
40. Lorig KR, Mazonson PD, Holman HR: Evidence suggesting that health education for self-management in patients with chronic arthritis has sustained health benefits while reducing health care costs. Arthritis Rheum. 1993;36:439–446.
41. Lorig K, Holman H, Sobel D, et al: *Living a Healthy Life with Chronic Conditions.* Boulder, CO, Bull Publishing, 2006.
42. Lorig KR, Sobel DS, Stewart AL, et al: Evidence suggesting that a chronic disease self-management program can improve health status while reducing hospitalization. Med Care. 1999;37:5–14.
43. Lorig KR, Ritter P, Stewart AL, et al: Chronic disease self-management program: 2-year health status and health care utilization outcomes. Med Care. 2001;39:1217–1223.
44. Griffin S, Kinmonth AL: Systems for routine surveillance for people with diabetes mellitus. Cochrane Database Syst Rev. 2000;(2):CD000541.
45. Norris SL, Lau J, Smith SJ, et al: Self-management education for adults with type 2 diabetes. Diabetes Care. 2002;25:1159–1171.
46. Diabetes Prevention Program Research Group: Reduction in the incidence of type 2 diabetes with lifestyle intervention or metformin. NEJM. 2002;346:393–403.
47. Gwadry-Sridhar FH, Flintoft V, Lee DS, et al: A systematic review and meta-analysis of studies comparing readmission rates and mortality rates in patients with heart failure. Arch Intern Med. 2004;164:2315–2320.
48. Holland R. Battersby J, Harvey I, et al: Systematic review of multidisciplinary interventions in heart failure. Heart. 2005;91:899–906.
49. McAlister FA, Lawson FME, Teo KK, et al: A systematic review of randomized trials of disease management programs in heart failure. Am J Med. 2001;110;378–384.
50. Wagner EH: Deconstructing heart failure disease management. Ann Intern Med. 2004;131:644–646.
51. Newman S, Steed L, Mulligan K: Self-management interventions for chronic illness. Lancet. 2004;364:1523–1537.

CHAPTER SIX

Improving Timely Access to Primary Care

Larry Waite had abdominal pain. After meals, a wave of cramps would spread across both lower quadrants. He experienced no diarrhea or vomiting. Calling his internist's office, he was told that the next available appointment was in 3 weeks; if his problem was urgent, he could go to the emergency department. Mr. Waite liked his internist and hated emergency departments. Once he spent 6 hours in an emergency department and came away with nothing more than a note telling him to contact his physician. Mr. Waite's pain continued for 3 weeks. Barely able to eat, he lost 8 pounds. When the appointment day arrived, his internist found an abdominal mass that proved to be a partially obstructing diverticular abscess.

Primary care practices have often failed to provide their patients with access to quality primary care at the time when the patient needs it [1]. Forty percent of emergency department visits are not urgent. Many take place because patients cannot obtain a prompt primary care appointment [2]. From 1997 to 2001, the percentage of people reporting an inability to obtain a timely appointment rose from 23% to 33% [3]. In 2001, 43% of adults reporting an urgent condition were sometimes unable to receive care as soon as they wanted [4]. A 2001 women's health survey found that 28% of women in fair or poor health reported delaying care or failing to receive care because of an inability to obtain a timely physician appointment [5]. In its landmark report *Crossing the Quality Chasm:*

A New Health System for the 21st Century, the Institute of Medicine designated *timeliness* as one of the six key *aims for improvement* in health care [6].

Overfilled appointment books create a state of disarray in primary care offices. Receptionists may spend 10 minutes on the telephone negotiating appointment times with patients, causing other patients to wait interminably on hold. As the day progresses, the stack of messages on the physician's desk—each requiring a chart to be pulled and later refiled—grows as patients insist on speaking with their physician. Medical assistants and nurses are mired in telephone triage, attempting to determine the urgency of patients' problems. Patients with urgent-sounding problems are squeezed in during lunch hours and into the early evening. The task of returning telephone calls to patients who were unable to schedule an appointment because of crammed schedules lengthens a physician's seemingly endless day. Upon instructing receptionists to reschedule a patient with diabetes in a month, physicians are called on the intercom and told that no slots are open at that time. One physician described the reception desk as a war zone with patients and receptionists battling over appointment times. It is hard to judge who is more stressed and dissatisfied—patient, receptionist, or physician.

THREE ACCESS MODELS FOR PRIMARY CARE

In response to this level of dysfunction, primary care practices utilize three distinct models of patient scheduling systems.

Traditional Model

The traditional model stratifies appointment demand into two streams: *urgent* and *nonurgent*. It strives to meet urgent demand today and nonurgent demand later. In this model, typically a patient contacts a receptionist, who determines the urgency of the clinical condition and checks with a nurse or physician for approval to bring patients who appear to be urgent into an already full schedule, often by double-booking an appointment slot. In many cases, the patient is sent elsewhere, usually to an emergency department.

The traditional model creates several problems. First, double-booking urgent patients creates shorter and thus less-productive visits with all patients, and heightens the stress on physicians. Second, the reduced time available for all patients, caused by double-booking urgent patients, often means that clinical issues are not dealt with and follow-up appointments are needed soon, thereby clogging up the appointment book even more. Third, a great deal of time of receptionists, medical assistants, nurses, and clinicians is wasted in trying to figure out what to do with patients whose problems need attention on the same day. Fourth, patients who are diverted to an emergency department are always told by the emergency physician to follow up with their primary care physician soon, thereby generating even more demand for appointments.

Carve-Out Model

Practices frequently seek relief from the traditional model by carving out a few slots each day for urgent visits. This carve-out model is far better than the traditional model, but fosters its own problems. One variety of the carve-out model designates one physician as *doc of the day*, with some slots open for urgent visits. Since in many cases the doc of the day is not the patient's personal physician, continuity of care is lost and the patient is often given an appointment with his or her own physician soon, again increasing demand and clogging appointment slots. Even if all physicians are given a few carve-out slots each day, that reduces their regular appointments and pushes nonurgent appointments even farther into the future. Moreover, phone triage systems often give nonurgent patients the urgent slots because patients—tired of waiting for appointments—justifiably make their complaints seem urgent.

In the case of both the traditional model and the carve-out model, nonurgent patients wait, often for weeks, for their appointment time to arrive. While waiting, they may get more sick, may go to the emergency department on their own, or may make frequent calls to the office, thereby creating pressures on the front desk.

Advanced Access Model

The advanced access model (also called open access or same-day scheduling) attempts to eliminate appointment delay [7–9]. Under this model, pioneered by Dr. Mark Murray, patients calling to see their physician are offered an appointment the same day. When a physician walks into the practice in the morning, one-half to two-thirds of his or her appointment slots are empty.

Primary care physicians, staff members, and managers cannot imagine having half-empty appointment books in a busy practice. However, one way to think about advanced access is: if a physician is seeing 25 patients per day and the patients made their appointments 6 weeks ago, why couldn't the physician see 25 patients per day and the patients made the appointments the same day?

No scheduling system, including advanced access, can work if a physician has too many patients. Patient demand for visits and physician capacity to schedule visits must be in balance. If demand permanently exceeds capacity, no system will work—neither the traditional model, the carve-out model, nor the advanced access model.

Advanced access does not sort patients into urgent and nonurgent categories; its message is to see all patients when they want to be seen. The motto of advanced access is *do today's work today*. Naturally, if patients do not want to be seen today, they should be given the choice to make an appointment in advance. However, if too many people make appointments in advance, the appointment books will be filled and advanced access will fail. Thus, the success of advanced access requires constant attention to the schedule and to the balancing of demand and capacity [8]. Advanced access can only work in a sustained way if patients are provided with alternatives to the face-to-face visit: phone, e-mail, or web-based care (see Chapter 7).

Katia has been the receptionist-in-charge of the front desk of Four-B family practice for 16 years. She is devoted to the practice, and is the person many patients—especially those who speak only Spanish—rely on to arrange their care. When one of the physicians returned from an Institute for Healthcare Improvement meeting and excitedly explained how the practice was going to move to advanced access, Katia was concerned. The patients can't all come the same day; the doctors will be here until 10 P.M. Besides, she makes sure that if people are really sick, they get prompt appointments. Other people can wait.

Rather than charge headlong into advanced access scheduling, the physicians first measured demand and capacity. The demand, calculated from a counting of all the patients who called for an appointment on a given day (external demand) plus all the patients for whom physicians made follow-up appointments (internal demand), was 90 visits a day.

Each day in the practice, three doctors were seeing 25 patients; thus the capacity was 75 visits a day. Either capacity had to grow or demand had to shrink.

Deciding that it was better to join the effort rather than to resist it, Katia became part of the improvement team working on advanced access. She adamantly opposed increasing capacity; the doctors were working too hard already. In fact, she wanted to reduce the daily appointment slots from 25 to 20, and suggested substituting phone advice for some of the visits. One of the doctors suggested launching a secure e-mail system to reduce face-to-face visits. Another idea was to try group visits, but Katia preferred not to change too many things too fast. The decision was made to change capacity to 60 visits, 30 phone advice calls, and e-mail visits for a small pilot group of patients to see how it affected the demand-capacity equation. Katia trained the front desk to suggest phone visits for patients with minor complaints and stable chronic disease follow-up. Before advanced access was even initiated, the new schedule was tried out for one physician to see how it worked. After a month, all physicians changed their schedules to 20 visits and 10 phone calls per day, and enough patients accepted the phone encounters to make the new system work. Now, supply and capacity were in balance at 90 encounters per day. It was time to move to advanced access.

Backlog Reduction

Busy primary care practices cannot start advanced access tomorrow. Their appointment books are already full, often for weeks ahead. The appointments already on the books are called the backlog. To achieve advanced access, the practice must eliminate the backlog that has accumulated.

If advanced access is implemented in a thoughtful manner, backlog reduction only happens once. Backlog reduction is a classic example of *no pain, no gain.* It requires a practice to see the patients who want an appointment the same day (so that future appointment slots will not keep getting filled) plus seeing the patients who already have appointments. The practice needs to add capacity temporarily through extra sessions, locum tenens, or extended work hours. A practice that sees 50 patients per day can eliminate a month-long backlog of future appointments by temporarily seeing an extra 50 patients per day for a month or 25 patients per day for 2 months. Ideally, a practice will substitute phone calls or e-mail interactions for face-to-face visits during the backlog reduction phase.

Access Measures

Advanced access must be data driven. Before implementing the reform, practice sites must know their daily demand for visits, capacity to provide appointments, and the availability of appointments.

The availability of appointments is tracked by following two metrics: third next available appointment and future open capacity. Third next available appointment measures the number of days a patient has to wait to get an appointment. The third next available physical examination is a sentinel marker. Physical examination is used rather than another appointment type because it is usually the latest scheduled. If access to physical examinations improves, all availability improves. The third appointment is featured because the first and second available appointments may reflect openings created by patients canceling appointments and thus does not accurately measure true accessibility. This measure is easily obtained, daily or weekly, by the receptionist counting the number of days until an opening for the third next physical examination appointment is on the schedule.

Future open capacity is the number of open appointment slots divided by the total number of appointment slots over the next 4 weeks. If a practice has 50 appointment slots per day, the denominator is 50 times 5 days/week times 4 weeks = 1000. In the traditional model, there might be 100 open slots during those 4 weeks, meaning a future open capacity of 10%. With advanced access, perhaps 600 of the appointment slots are still open, meaning that future open capacity is 60%. Generally, future open capacity of 60% or higher is a reasonable goal for the advanced access model. Practices with many elderly and chronically ill patients have a difficult time achieving a future open capacity of 60% since many appointments are scheduled in advance as follow-ups.

Continuity of Care

Advanced access attempts to preserve continuity of care. Under traditional appointment systems, patients may see an unfamiliar physician even if their own physician is present because the regular physician's appointment slots are full. The new model can improve continuity because all physicians have appointment slots available.

Many primary care physicians do not work every day. A patient calling to request an appointment with a physician not present that day should be given the choice of seeing another physician today or waiting to schedule an appointment with his or her physician later in the week. The patient can then balance the value of continuity of care against the competing value of immediate access.

The Four-B advanced access improvement team decided that offering same-day appointments to all patients might be unrealistic. For one thing, since the physicians saw patients 4 days each week, a patient's physician may not be present the day a patient calls. They set their goal—100% of appointments would be offered within 3 days of the patient's call. They set up a run chart to track their progress, using the metrics of the third next available appointment and future open capacity. They also decided to measure continuity of care, which is the percentage of total visits that are visits to the patient's personal physician.

The baseline data showed a third next available appointment of 30 days for one physician, 40 days for two other physicians, and 60 days for the fourth physician. The future open capacity for the entire practice was 7% for the next 4 weeks. The continuity of care measure was 70%.

The improvement team decided to work down the backlog over 2 months by increasing the length of the workday for all physicians and by persuading as many patients as possible to have telephone visits. Patients calling for new appointments were either given face-to-face appointments the same week or phone visits the same day. Many opted for the phone, which helped the backlog reduction process. Physicians grumbled that they were staying until 9 P.M. talking to patients by phone, but after 2 weeks the access metrics were already improving.

Two months after day zero the third next available appointment was less than 10 days for all the physicians and the future open capacity for the practice was 50%. Three weeks later, third next available was 5 days for all but one physician.

Katia was put in charge of keeping these metrics at the goals of 5 days for third next available appointment and 60% for future open capacity. She also tracked continuity of care, which had remained about the same at 70%. When she saw the third next available appointment rising, she asked the receptionists to make extra efforts to persuade patients to utilize the telephone visit option. In addition, the physicians, who used to see their patients with chronic illnesses every month, were telling those patients to make a phone appointment each month and—unless the illness deteriorated—a face-to-face appointment every 3 months, thereby reducing internal demand.

A year later, the Four Bs were still achieving their advanced access goals. The sustained success depended on constant attention by Katia to tweak demand and capacity.

Demand Reduction

A busy primary care practice needs to reduce visit demand in order to sustain advanced access. This can be done in several ways:

- Make return visits less frequent for stable patients. Many return-visit intervals became conventional years ago, without evidence of their effect on clinical outcomes [10].

- Reduce the scope of the physician's responsibilities by developing and training a care team such that nonphysicians can do routine chronic and preventive care (see Chapters 4 and 9).

- Use the telephone and electronic communication for medical encounters that do not need a face-to-face visit (see Chapter 7).

- For the small percentage of patients in any practice who utilize a disproportionate amount of practice resources (frequent users), make a plan for each of those patients that utilizes outside resources and nonphysician caregiver time to address the patient's concerns without frequent and lengthy physician visits.

It is true that personnel in many practices are busy all the time and cannot take on additional work. However, an analysis of how practice staff spends their time will often uncover waste that can be eliminated. Advanced access itself can reduce waste; by offering all patients an appointment within a few days, advanced access virtually eliminates the triage function, freeing up personnel for other tasks, and reducing interruptions and telephone callbacks. The rate of *no-shows* goes down since patients making an appointment for the same day or same week rarely fail to come [11]. No-shows are wasteful because personnel are engaged in making appointments, pulling charts, and evaluating whether the patient who did not come needs proactive follow-up.

Moreover, some systems who have successfully implemented advanced access (Table 6-1) have found that patient demand decreases because patients are more often able to see their own clinician [9].

Panel Size

Patient demand is determined by panel size and panel composition. In a capitated primary care practice, a physician's panel size is the number of patients enrolled to that physician. In fee-for-service and mixed practices, it is defined as all patients seen by a physician in the past 18 months (12 months appear to undercount, and 24 months overcount panel size).

TABLE 6–1

Advice from the expert

Mark Murray initially conceived of advanced access and has helped many practices improve their access. Here is some of Dr. Murray's advice [12].

How should we start?

Create a team to address the problem. Measure supply and demand and make sure they balance. Advanced access will not be sustainable if demand for appointments exceeds capacity to offer appointments.

What if a physician's demand exceeds her capacity—if she is overpaneled?

Her panel needs to be reduced, or she needs another clinician to share her panel with. If this is not done, the entire practice will be playing catch-up with her patients' needs.

How do we reduce our backlog of already scheduled appointments?

The only way is to do extra work (lunch hours, working late) and to make return-visit intervals as long as possible consistent with high-quality care. Display data, showing reduced waiting times, to show that the effort is working.

What about appointments that need to be prescheduled?

If demand equals capacity, most practices can preschedule patients and still have plenty of appointment slots open. Prescheduled appointments should be late in the week or early in the day, when demand is lower. Practices with many older patients or newborns will have a higher proportion of prescheduled appointments.

What if we fail?

Failure is usually due to a leadership problem, lack of constant measurement and review of the data, or imbalance between demand and capacity.

Panel composition refers to the percentage of patients in a panel who are elderly and chronically ill; the higher that percentage, the greater the demand. Given an average patient panel, not overly weighted with elderly and chronically ill people, about 0.7% to 0.8% of the panel will call for an appointment on an average day [7]. For a panel of 2500, this means 17–20 daily calls. For panels with high-risk patients, demand rises markedly—a reality that limits the utility of measuring panel size to predict demand.

Contingency Plans

Contingency plans are needed to keep supply and demand in balance on a daily basis, despite inevitable variations in either. Scheduling algorithms that work well most of the time will fail under special circumstances; such circumstances require plan B [8].

Demand for appointments increases at such times as back-to-school physicals, influenza season, the day after Thanksgiving, and the days following clinician vacations. Capacity declines when clinicians are away on vacation or continuing medical education. Contingency plans are needed to keep supply and demand in balance during those periods. Practices can predict variations in demand and capacity and respond. For example, Mondays are the heaviest days; thus, few prescheduled appointments should be made after 10 A.M. on Monday. More clinicians should be scheduled to see patients at the time of back-to-school physicals and flu season. Sometimes, third next available appointment will increase by a few days, in which case the practice must do all possible to bring it back down quickly. Once appointment books start filling up again, the gains of advanced access can be squandered.

CASE STUDIES OF ADVANCED ACCESS

Much can be learned from anecdotal descriptions of organizations implementing this reform. The following section contains descriptions of some real-world experiences with advanced access [9]. Seven actual cases are described—four that successfully implemented advanced access, followed by three with less success. (The successful organizations are named, the less successful are not.)

Highland Family Practice

Highland Family Practice, a private fee-for-service medical office in rural Virginia with two physicians and a nurse practitioner, cares for a wide variety of patients, 20% of whom are elderly or disabled. The practice has used advanced access scheduling since it opened in 2000. Each physician has a patient panel exceeding 1500 and sees an average of 28 patients per day. Given their broad scope of practice (including obstetrics and office procedures), the panels are reaching their limit. At the beginning of an average day, from 30% to 50% of appointment slots are open. Elderly patients and those with long-term conditions are offered prescheduled appointments, but these are not made on Mondays or near holidays. Some days are too busy and the physicians stay late; other days are comfortable, with eight to ten patients per physician per half-day. The physicians like advanced access because they are not double-booking patients into already full schedules.

Demand is measured daily by a receptionist who counts the number of calls for appointments, physician-generated follow-up appointments, and drop-ins. These measures help the physicians predict how demand is increasing as the practice grows and how demand varies with days of the week and seasons of the year. Provider capacity is matched with the demand projections with the goal to *stay ahead of the demand curve*. Although the management of advanced access does consume time and energy, it saves the energy wasted in traditional scheduling systems that require constant juggling of schedules, making triage decisions, and answering telephone calls interrupting patient visits. Advanced access has been sustained through 2005; the two physician owners of the practice are committed to the concept for their patients and for themselves.

South Central Foundation

In the past, 85% of care for patients in the South Central Foundation, the primary care system of the Alaska Native Medical Center in Anchorage, Alaska, was delivered in urgent care settings. Waits during acute visits were many hours long, and waiting times for nonurgent appointments were measured in months. Only a few patients could identify their own clinician and even fewer saw their clinician of choice.

Currently, patients in this system have a guarantee of a same-day appointment, usually with their own physician, if they call before 4 P.M. A great majority see their own clinician. Managerial staff have linked each patient with a specific physician, reduced the appointment backlog, developed contingency plans for vacations and other expected events, reduced demand by encouraging continuity of care, and transferred to care managers some work previously performed by physicians.

As of November 2004, 60% of appointment slots in the family medicine clinic were unfilled at 8 A.M. each morning, allowing same day access to function. This achievement has been sustained for at least 4 years. One key to success has been a reduction in demand; the number of primary care physician visits per enrolled patient dropped by 40% from 2000 to 2005. This was accomplished by an increase in visits to nonphysician team members.

Backlog reduction took several months, and physicians were initially skeptical but survived the process with encouragement from management. Moving to advanced access often highlights other system problems. For example, telephones functioned poorly, which prevented patients from calling for same-day appointments and prompted a board member to tell the management, "You gave me the Mercedes but forgot to give me the keys." This bottleneck has been corrected. Since patients can come the same day if they call before 4 P.M., the end of the day can be burdensome to clinicians.

This practice has been successful because its management devotes a great deal of effort in solving problems as they arise, includes the entire staff in the process, utilizes data systems to track access measures, and has sought assistance from outside experts experienced in implementing advanced access.

Central DuPage Physician Group

A primary care network with multiple sites in the western suburbs of Chicago, Illinois, this physician group launched advanced access in July 2001. The majority of patients are privately insured with 23% insured with Medicare and 2% insured with Medicaid. Most primary care physicians work full time—32 clinical hours per week—and see about 25 patients per day. Prior to advanced access, the third next available physical examination for some physicians was more than 35 days. A carve-out system was tried, but pressure to fill the frozen slots early was irresistible.

After 4–6 weeks of backlog reduction, access ranged from 0–3 days, where it remained. Patient satisfaction rose from the 72nd to the 85th percentile of a standardized, national survey, and continuity of care (percentage of patient visits taking place with their own physician) increased from 40% to 75%.

Though physician panels were not excessive (average 1800), backlog reduction was difficult; some physicians worked extra shifts while others stayed late in the evenings. After the backlog was eliminated, schedules had to be managed daily to solve problems, particularly for the more popular physicians. Under the new model, some physicians work harder while others work less. As the executive director explained, "To sustain the gains after working down the backlog is not a slam dunk."

Bellevue Hospital

The outpatient department of Bellevue Hospital in New York, a large urban public teaching hospital, started advanced access in some primary care and specialty clinics in July 2001. The third next available appointment prior to that date was in the vicinity of 12 weeks; by July 2002 the figure had dropped to 1–3 days for primary care, human immunodeficiency virus, neurology, and geriatrics clinics. Patient satisfaction improved by 25%.

The champion of the new model has been the medical director, who first attempted the change in 1999 but failed. At that time, a major obstacle was the rotation of residents through the clinics to such an extent that 80% of physicians were part-timers. The medical director succeeded in changing the system, increasing the number of full-time physicians. For part-time rotating residents, teams were established with a full-time non-physician serving as the team anchor. The scheduling reform, together with the medical director's tireless persuasion of countless people in the institution, enabled the second attempt to succeed. Other public hospitals are currently working to emulate this improvement in access for the nation's lowest-income patients [11].

As of early 2006, the waiting time for appointments had risen because budget cutbacks made it impossible to handle the phone volume required in a same-day scheduling system. The hospital is continuing to make primary care improvements that are likely to result in another reduction in waiting times. Bellevue's experience demonstrates that advanced access is a sustainable improvement only as part of a multifaceted improvement effort.

Practice A: A Small University-Based Practice

The medical director of this practice returned from a meeting at which advanced access was presented, excited about the concept. A committee of clinicians and administrators was assembled to initiate the innovation. However, the six key changes—balancing supply and demand, working down the backlog, reducing appointment types, developing contingency plans, reducing demand, and increasing capacity—were neither put into practice nor was a model for organizational change adopted. The innovation never moved from planning to the implementation stage and the reform withered.

Practice B: An Integrated Delivery System

A health system in a medium-sized city launched advanced access at some primary care sites. In one site, the third next available appointment for some physicians was 40 days. The backlog was reduced and advanced access was achieved. However, some physicians left and demand increased due to the closing of another nearby primary care site. With this mismatch of demand and capacity, access deteriorated. The site returned to a carve-out system.

In another primary care site in the same system, most physicians never embraced the idea, thinking that the reform was being pushed by administrators for the purpose of increasing market share. Most physicians were part-timers, had hospital as well as ambulatory care duties, and were used to maintaining tight control over their schedules. The site has had difficulty obtaining outpatient charts from the hospital's medical records department, making the physicians wary that same-day appointments would result in even fewer available charts. Due to this combination of real system constraints and resistance to change, the site never made a serious attempt at advanced access.

Practice C: A Community Health Center

A community health center serving a low-income urban population attempted to initiate advanced access, but did so in a rigid manner. The health center made it difficult for patients to obtain prescheduled appointments by requiring most of them to call by telephone on the day they wished to come. The telephone system became so overburdened that many patients were unable to call. Although access improved for those patients able to be seen promptly, access diminished for other patients. Clinicians became concerned that elderly and disabled people appeared less able to navigate the new system. This example reveals that advanced access must be implemented in a flexible manner, attuned to the particular needs of each institution and its patients. Some patients—the chronically ill and children with special needs—fare better with prescheduled appointments. Advanced access is not meant to punish patients by restricting prescheduled appointments that some patients prefer or need.

Lessons of the Case Studies

Practices that successfully implemented the advanced access model measured their demand and capacity and developed contingency plans to match capacity and demand daily. When asked if the energy needed to sustain the advanced access model was burdensome, one physician responded, "It is far less effort than handling the daily triage and double-booking chaos of the old system." Most practices reported that managerial time is needed on a permanent basis to sustain advanced access. In order to increase capacity, some successful practices have created team structures to delegate some tasks, formerly performed by physicians, to other practice staff. All practices had trouble working down the backlog—a problem especially difficult in larger organizations when advanced access was introduced as a management-generated rather than a physician-generated concept—with the goal of increasing patient satisfaction and market share. Because the benefits of advanced access come more quickly for management (decreasing appointment delay) than for physicians (a less stressful workday), motivating employed physicians to undertake this innovation is not easy. Advanced access is more easily accomplished in smaller private offices and when it is initiated by physicians who are owners of the practice, and are therefore motivated to reduce hassles created by denying patients prompt appointments.

The practices that did not succeed in implementing advanced access stumbled for a variety of reasons. Practice A never moved beyond the necessary task of working down the backlog. Practice B achieved initial success, only to have the model falter when confronted with abrupt and unexpected changes in supply and demand. Practice C encountered fundamental problems in managing telephone demand and in flexibly balancing internal and external visit demand from a vulnerable patient population.

Physicians invariably mention two characteristics as essential to achieving and sustaining advanced access: (1) the willingness of the majority of physicians to make a major change in their mode of functioning, and (2) ongoing administrative support and leadership.

RESEARCH ON ADVANCED ACCESS

Research on advanced access is in its infancy. As more and more practices experiment with this model, more studies can be expected.

HealthPartners Medical Group in Minnesota studied its experience in introducing advanced access at 17 of its primary care clinics. Two years after advanced access was launched, the average time to third next available appointment had dropped from 18 to 4 days. One hundred and ten interviews with physicians, managers, and other clinic staff revealed that the most successful clinics had strong leadership and cohesive teamwork with meetings and productive communication. While advanced access created tensions among physicians, they tended to support the change because the appointment process had been broken previously [13].

A family practice residency program implemented advanced access for one faculty-resident team and retained the traditional appointment system for the other team. Prior to the innovation, waiting times were similar for the two teams, while 1 year later the advanced access team's third next available appointment was 5 days compared with 21 days for the traditional team. Continuity of care improved for the advanced access team but not for the traditional team. Panel size was somewhat higher for the advanced access team. While the residents in the advanced access team were more satisfied than prior to the innovation, patient satisfaction was not significantly different between the two teams [14].

Six British practices having two to nine physicians, which had introduced advanced access, were studied. The average time to get an appointment prior to the implementation of advanced access was 10 days, declining to under 2 days after implementation. Panel sizes varied from 1800 to 3400 per full-time general practitioner. The research team interviewed physicians, managers, and receptionists. Receptionists were positive toward the innovation; whereas they had previously battled patients over appointment times, advanced access allowed them to fulfill patients' needs. They no longer had to triage patients into urgent and nonurgent, which had created considerable work stress. Managers also liked advanced access, which reduced bureaucratic work, cut down patient complaints, and lowered the stress level in the practice. Physicians had mixed feelings about advanced access. They appreciated the improved satisfaction of patients, but complained that they had more work and spent more time in the office than before. The physicians also felt that continuity of care had declined after the institution of advanced access because patients often preferred to be seen the same day, whether or not their personal physician was available [15].

CONFRONTING PROBLEMS

Dr. Aretha Love, a family physician, is very popular with her patients. Whereas the other seven physicians in her practice have panels of 1600–1800 patients, her panel exceeds 2500 patients, many with chronic conditions. After finally eliminating her backlog, she was pleased to find that 50% of her appointments were open each day. However, she received an average of 24 telephone requests for appointments each day, with only 12 open slots. Although she attempted to do today's work today, her backlog was reaccumulating. Her future open capacity sank to 15%. Dr. Love did not want to return to the old way, but she could not sustain the new way. She demanded a meeting with the practice administrator.

Sustaining advanced access after eliminating the backlog is an active daily process. What tools could practices use to help overpaneled physicians, like Dr. Love, whose demand exceeds her capacity? The administrator and Dr. Love first agreed to protect her from some obvious sources of excessive demand for visits. Dr. Love's schedule was closed to new patients not already in her patient panel. She would no longer see patients of other physicians on days when her colleagues were not working or on vacation. The administrator and Dr. Love, acknowledging the relative undersupply of clinician resources for Dr. Love's panel, agreed to transfer an underutilized nurse practitioner from another site to form a care team with her. In addition, the practice administrator realized that he needed to manage schedules more actively. He assigned a designated staff scheduler to work with all physicians' schedules on a daily basis in order to match demand and capacity. Schedules for all physicians were to be kept largely empty on Mondays (when demand is greatest) and during the week following a vacation. Similar contingency planning would be done for periods of increased demand such as during the influenza season. Finally, Dr. Love and the practice administrator embarked on some innovative strategies to redesign the care process. A nurse or medical assistant—no longer needed to perform triage functions—would be trained to assist Dr. Love in routine follow-up visits for patients with stable hypertension and diabetes. The practice would determine which patients on her panel were frequent utilizers and arrange for care managers, family members, or home care nurses to assist in their care, in order to reduce their demand on her time. Dr. Love would also be assisted in arranging a weekly group medical visit allowing her to see 15 patients in a 2-hour period.

Dr. Sandra Wise was not convinced. After hearing about the success of the new model at the pediatric site of her practice, some of her internal medicine colleagues wanted to try it. Dr. Wise resisted. "My panel has chronically ill, elderly patients. My diabetics need to come each month. My heart failure patients need to come regularly. My schedule is filled with prebooked appointments. This is not for me."

Dr. Wise has a point; physicians with many patients with chronic illness have trouble guarding white space on their appointment books.

Some practices solve Dr. Wise's problem by making *pending appointments*—asking them to call for a follow-up visit in, for example, 2 months. Rather than penciling the appointment into the appointment book, the date of the pending appointment is entered into a computer or tickler file so that the patient can be sent a reminder. Such a system avoids filled appointment books while preventing patients with long-term illnesses from falling between the cracks. Some physicians succeed in keeping 50% of their appointments open; those with large panels of elderly patients or newborns have more appointments booked in advance.

The advanced access model has a potentially symbiotic relationship to the Chronic Care Model, described in Chapter 4. Patients with chronic illness should be followed up with planned visits, performed by non-physician care managers under physician-created protocols, thereby reducing demand for prescheduled physician appointment slots and help-ing to match demand and capacity. At the same time, the advanced access model allows patients with an acute exacerbation of their illness to have prompt access to their own physician.

A number of questions about advanced access have not been answered with definitive research studies. Should elderly patients with certain diagnoses be encouraged to request same-day appointments or should they be scheduled in advance? Are certain patient panel character-istics inappropriate for the new model? Does improved access for some types of patients potentially come at the expense of diminished access for others? Does advanced access reduce delays in a manner that actually improves clinical outcomes, such as more rapid recovery from acute ill-nesses and avoidance of exacerbations of chronic conditions? Are physi-cians working shorter or longer hours under advanced access, and how does physician stress impact the sustainability of the model? Can advanced access be sustained over many years, or will it wither, as enthu-siasm for the novel is no longer a major motivation for the reform?

HOW TO BEGIN

Timely access to primary care is a problem for many patients. Primary care practices must become more innovative in designing new scheduling models to resolve this problem. In an era calling for creativity and experi-mentation in primary care, the advanced access model is one approach to reforming basic scheduling procedures [16]. Some practices will not choose advanced access as their goal; they would prefer to work with a carve-out system or a modified advanced access model that attempts to *do this week's work this week rather than do today's work today.*

Primary care practices with access problems can take some initial steps to evaluate their potential for improving access. The first step begins with collecting baseline data on demand, capacity, panel size, continuity rates, and each physician's third next available appointment. Most offices and clinics can readily measure these indicators using existing scheduling templates and staffing records and by monitoring calls for appointments. Once baseline data are collected, the practice must assess whether capacity is sufficient to satisfy visit demand. This assessment involves examination of not only overall demand and supply, but also of daily and seasonal fluctuations in demand and supply that create scheduling bottlenecks. Practices not ready to immerse themselves in an advanced access model may take the smaller steps of initiating incremental reforms in scheduling, such as planning more systematically for staffing contingencies like vacations, rethinking triage procedures, and redesigning routine office visits to make more effective use of clinician time.

Practices that do choose advanced access as their goal need to realize that advanced access will fail without redesign of the face-to-face 15-minute physician visit syndrome. Most practices need to reduce visit demand by instituting nonphysician care management for patients with chronic conditions and phone or electronic encounters where appropriate.

Before taking the plunge into advanced access, it is important for primary care practices to hold serious discussions about their desire to undertake this reform. It is natural for the human mind to push today's work off until tomorrow. Advanced access requires that physicians begin to think in a new way—pull tomorrow's work into today.

REFERENCES

1. Goitein M: Waiting patiently. N Engl J Med. 1990;323:604–608.
2. Cunningham PJ, Clancy CM, Cohen JW, et al: The use of hospital emergency departments for nonurgent health problems: a national perspective. Med Care Res Rev. 1995;52:453–474.
3. Strunk BC, Cunningham PJ. *Treading Water: Americans' Access to Needed Medical Care, 1997-2001.* Washington, DC, Center for Studying Health System Change, March 2002.

4. Greenblatt J: *Access to Urgent Medical Care, 2001*. Rockville, MD, Agency for Healthcare Research and Quality, 2002. Statistical brief No. 08.

5. Women's Health in the United States: *Health Coverage and Access to Care*. Menlo Park, CA, Kaiser Family Foundation, May 2002.

6. Institute of Medicine: *Crossing the Quality Chasm: A New Health System for the 21st Century*. Washington, DC, National Academy Press, 2001.

7. Murray M, Tantau C: Same-day appointments: exploding the access paradigm. Fam Pract Manag. 2000;7:45–50.

8. Murray M, Berwick DM: Advanced access: reducing waiting and delays in primary care. JAMA. 2003;289:1035–1040.

9. Murray M, Bodenheimer T, Rittenhouse D, et al: Improving timely access to primary care: case studies of the advanced access model. JAMA. 2003;289:1042–1046.

10. Schwartz L, Woloshin S, Wasson J, et al: Setting the revisit interval in primary care. J Gen Intern Med. 1999;14:230–235.

11. Singer IA: *Advanced Access: A New Paradigm in the Delivery of Ambulatory Care Services*. Washington, DC, National Association of Public Hospitals and Health Systems, 2001.

12. Murray M: Answers to your questions about same-day scheduling. Fam Pract Manag. 2005;12(3):59-64. (*www.aafp.org/fpm/20050300/59answ.html*)

13. Solberg LI, Hroscikoski MC, Sperl-Hillen JM, et al: Key issues in transforming health care organizations for quality: the case of advanced access. Jt Comm J Qual Saf. 2004;30:15–24.

14. Belardi FG, Weir S, Craig FW: A controlled trial of an advanced access appointment system in a residency family medicine center. Fam Med. 2004;36:341–345.

15. Ahluwalia S, Offredy M: A qualitative study of the impact of the implementation of advanced access in primary healthcare on the working lives of general practice staff. BMC Fam Pract. 2005, 6:39–70.

16. (*www.ihi.org/IHI/Topics/OfficePractices/Access/*)

CHAPTER SEVEN

Alternatives to the 15-minute Visit

One morning, Dr. Ivan Rushakoff was running from room to room, seeing one patient after another, frustrated by the frenzied atmosphere of each visit. Dr. Rushakoff's disgruntlement was exceeded only by the discontent of the patients. "There has to be a better way," fumed the doctor. "Each patient sits isolated in a room behind closed doors waiting for my late entry and hurried exit. Not only that, most of the patients have similar medical problems." A mental light bulb illuminated in Dr. Rushakoff's brain, "Why don't I see them all together?"

The fictional Dr. Rushakoff's discovery mirrors the actual birth of the chronic care group visit. Dr. John Scott, a primary care physician at the Kaiser Permanente facility at Wheat Ridge, Colorado, frustrated with the tyranny of the 15-minute one-on-one visit, conceived of and implemented the group visit idea in 1991.

Since John Scott's innovation, the group visit concept has branched out into three distinct varieties: the Cooperative Health Care Clinic (Dr. Scott's model), the specialty group visit, and the Drop-In Group Medical Appointment. All three were pioneered at Kaiser Permanente practices.

Group visits are not the only alternative to the traditional patient visit. Telephone care, remote telemedicine, e-mail, and web-based encounters are growing in importance. Low-tech group visits expand the range of human interactions in primary care. Technology-based telephonic and electronic encounters promote convenient and efficient clinician-patient communication.

GROUP VISITS

The Cooperative Health Care Clinic

John Scott's Cooperative Health Care Clinic model is an alternative, not an add-on, to individual physician visits [1]. Patients choosing the group model see their physician during a once-a-month group session. If they need more physician time, they can also make an individual physician appointment, but generally the group visit is the way in which they receive their primary care. This model emphasizes continuity of care; the same patients attend their physician's group month after month. Dr. Scott has some patients who have been seeing him in group visits for over 10 years.

The Cooperative Health Care Clinic model targets elderly people who are chronically ill, but not frail. Those who are hearing impaired or demented cannot participate in groups. Otherwise, virtually all diagnoses are accepted. The group of 15–20 patients, sitting around a large table, first receives a brief educational talk about a health problem. While the nurse performs blood pressures, blood sugars, diabetic foot exams, and other functions, the physician goes around the room taking focused histories and whatever portions of physical exams are needed and appropriate in a group setting. Patients are referred to physical therapy, specialty care, or dietary counseling as needed, prescriptions are written, plans are made for the management of each problem, and the physician charts the visit into the Kaiser Permanente (Colorado) electronic medical record. Some patients call others during the month to see how they are getting along. For those few patients who need privacy for a sensitive discussion or physical exam, the physician schedules time following the group session.

As the physician is directing attention to one patient, the others may listen, talk quietly with one another, or chime in with their suggestions and experiences. Dr. Scott recounts: "I was talking about arthritis one time, and a little voice in the back of the room said: 'You mean I'm going to have to live with this? How am I going to live with this?' Another woman held up a disfigured rheumatoid hand and said, 'Honey, at the break I'll tell you how.' "

At an actual Kaiser Permanente (Colorado) group visit in December 2000, the physician group leader asked the patients "Do you know what 'high risk' means?" One man piped up: "If you are about to lay down and die you are high risk." During that group session, the physician—with the other patients listening—adjusted the medications of one patient whose blood pressure was 150/112. One patient wanted to know the pros and cons of back surgery for a herniated lumbar disc; two other patients—one treated with surgery and one without—recounted their experiences. A patient wanted the results of a recent shoulder x-ray; the physician accessed the information on the computer, showed it to the group, and discussed the patient's treatment options. Another patient wanted her lipid results; the ensuing discussion interested the entire group.

The group visit ended with a 20-minute intense meeting between the physician, a patient with amyotrophic lateral sclerosis (ALS), and the patient's family. The discussion centered on the possible need for a permanent feeding tube since the patient was beginning to aspirate his food. The patient and family had given permission for other patients in the group to be part of the meeting. After the discussion, another patient remarked "I thought I had a problem, but after hearing this, I have nothing to complain about."

Kaiser Permanente (Colorado) has organized 40 groups similar to Dr. Scott's. Both physicians and patients groups are voluntary. Physicians are trained in conducting groups and are mentored until they feel comfortable. Not only do group visits allow patients to help each other, they also give patients the feeling that they are spending adequate time with their physician. Even though each patient may receive only 5–10 minutes of the physician's individual attention, they experience being in the room with the physician for 90 minutes.

Disease-Specific Group Visits

Brian Able, physician assistant, has organized two series of group visits for patients with diabetes at Pioneer Community Health Center in rural Georgia. The visits consist of an interactive educational session, diabetes management for each participant, and goal setting. One series is conducted in English, the other in Spanish. For the six weekly group meetings, the educational topics cover the nature of diabetes, diet, exercise, home glucose testing, medications, and foot care. The team leading the visits includes PA Able, a dietician, a medical assistant, and a patient with diabetes who has become a successful self-manager.

Prior to the meeting, the medical assistant has collected the clinical data on each patient, and after the 30-minute educational session she informs each patient which tests or eye referrals are due, and gives them any necessary paperwork. Meanwhile, PA Able makes medication adjustments for each patient, with other patients often chiming in. If a patient newly requires insulin, patients already taking insulin give advice. The medical assistant leads the group's goal setting (see Chapter 5); patients talk about how they did on their action plans from the previous week, problem solve, and make revised action plans. A buddy system encourages pairs of patients to call one another during the week to problem-solve difficulties.

At the end of the final session, the harmony of the group is disrupted as several patients object that the group only has six sessions and demand that the group continue on a permanent basis.

Group visits, based on the John Scott model, bring together patients with a variety of diagnoses into one group. In another type of group visit, the participants have the same chronic condition: diabetes, hypertension, arthritis, fibromyalgia, or congestive heart failure. Disease-specific group visits can also join patients with a cluster of related conditions, such as diabetes, hypertension, elevated cholesterol, and other cardiac risk factors.

Some disease-specific groups limit themselves to patient education and behavior-change counseling; these are add-ons to the individual clinician-patient visit. More innovative are groups that take the place of the traditional visit by including the entire management of the disease including the prescribing of medications.

Because few primary care practices have the resources to provide group visits to the large numbers of chronically ill patients who could benefit, groups are often limited to a few sessions, thereby allowing a new set of patients to attend the group the next time it is offered. A practice goal—borrowing from the John Scott groups—might be to offer permanent disease-specific groups that take the place of individual visits for interested patients. Some practices are also experimenting with group visits for prenatal care and well-child care, and for other types of encounters for which a group experience may be both beneficial to patients and efficient for the practice.

Drop-In Group Medical Appointments

In 1996, Edward Noffsinger, a clinical psychologist, developed the concept of the Drop-In Group Medical Appointment (DIGMA) at Kaiser Permanente's Santa Teresa facility in San Jose, California. In contrast to John Scott's continuity model—in which the same patients attend their clinician's group for years—DIGMAs have different patients each time. Patients may call in advance or simply drop in [2].

DIGMAs generally run for 60–90 minutes with a census of 12–20 patients. They may be conducted by primary care physicians, mixing patients with a variety of diagnoses, or by specialists concentrating on one diagnosis. The initial DIGMAs piloted at Kaiser Permanente were led by physicians in primary care, oncology, neurology, and rheumatology. In Dr. Noffsinger's model, groups are led by a physician, a behavioral health specialist, and nursing staff.

Although the Cooperative Health Care Clinic model emphasizes improved quality and financial savings, DIGMA's main benefit is improved access. Rather than having receptionists squeeze into a physician's filled schedule patients requesting visits on a semiurgent basis, they can add these patients into a weekly DIGMA. DIGMAs dovetail perfectly with same-day access scheduling (see Chapter 6), enabling physicians to see two or three times more patients than individual appointments would allow. As with John Scott's groups, physician leaders have time, following the DIGMA, to see individually patients who need privacy. Patients must always be given the choice of a DIGMA or an individual physician visit.

A 2001 DIGMA taking place at the Palo Alto Medical Foundation in Northern California involved about 20 patients. Two patients needed blood pressure medications changed and four patients with diabetes needed diet and medication adjustments to improve their blood sugars. As in all group visits, patients in DIGMAs help one another. One poorly controlled diabetic patient refused to take insulin in spite of numerous entreaties by his physician; at the DIGMA another person with diabetes remarked, "you remind me of myself before I had my first amputation." The patient started insulin. Two patients with fibromyalgia had suggestions for one another. For a patient with acute back pain, the physician did a history and brief physical exam in front of the group; then others with back pain gave advice regarding spine classes, home exercises, and other treatment modalities. One patient wanted a drug for weight reduction and instead received a 5-minute educational discussion from the physician with other patients adding their experiences.

Other Types of Group Visits

Care provided in groups has a long history in the health system and the larger community. Alcoholics Anonymous has provided a model for group therapy of addictive behaviors. Commercial and nonprofit diet programs take place in groups. Group psychotherapy has been conducted for decades. Yoga classes and exercise programs are group activities. The Chronic Disease Self-Management Program (see Chapter 5) brings together people with multiple chronic conditions. Because these other types of group visits do not generally take place in primary care sites, they are not covered in this chapter. However, primary care practices can create a list of group activities existing in their community and refer patients to these groups.

Research on Group Visits

In a large randomized controlled trial of John Scott's model with 24 months of follow-up, group visit patients had fewer hospital admissions, emergency visits, and professional services than usual care patients, leading to lower costs of $41.80 per member per month. Group visit patients reported higher satisfaction with their physician, better quality of life, and greater self-efficacy. It should be noted that all patients in the study, those randomized to group visits and to usual care, had expressed interest in attending the group visits; thus, there was no reason to suspect that the group visit patients were more motivated than the control patients [1, 3].

A randomized controlled trial of low-income patients, comparing group diabetes visits versus usual care, found that 76% of group visit participants completed at least 9 out of 10 recommended diabetes management processes (e.g., Hb A1c, foot exams, urine microalbumin) compared with 23% of control patients. During the brief time period of the study, no significant differences in glycemic or lipid control were found [4].

Another randomized controlled trial of diabetes group visits versus usual care was conducted in Italy. After 2 years, Hb A1c levels were significantly lower and HDL (high-density lipoprotein) cholesterol values were significantly higher for group visit patients than for patients receiving usual care. There was a tendency for group visit patients to have lower BMIs (body mass index). Physicians spent less time overall seeing 9–10 patients in a group, but patients had longer interaction with health care providers [5].

A third randomized controlled trial of diabetes group visits took place at Kaiser Permanente's Northern California Pleasanton facility. The visits combined patient education with clinical management. Group visit patients lowered Hb A1c levels by 1.3% compared with a reduction of 0.2% for patients receiving usual care. Group visit patients had reduced outpatient and hospital utilization and greater satisfaction with their care [6].

A Cochrane review performed a meta-analysis of group diabetes self-management training. The 11 studies reviewed generally involved patient education in groups rather than full-spectrum group visits, which also include medication management. Compared with usual care, group-based diabetes education was associated with reduced Hb A1c levels and a reduced need for diabetes medication [7].

Controlled trials of DIGMAs have not been reported. Physicians have testified that the number of phone calls and double-booked appointment slots drop when they offer DIGMAs. If a physician sees 6 individual patients in 90 minutes but 12 patients in a 90-minute DIGMA, costs might go down in capitated systems and reimbursements might increase under fee-for-service.

Obstacles to the Spread of Group Visits

Group visit models have begun to spread across the United States, appearing in some integrated delivery systems, academic medical centers, community health centers, public hospitals/health systems, and a few private primary care practices. In the case of both Cooperative Health Care Clinic and DIGMA models, an efficient administrative and scheduling infrastructure must be in place to manage the groups. In order to fulfill the business case for group visits, physicians should be able to see, and bill for, more people in the group setting than they would have seen as individual visits in the same time period. If the group census is not adequate, the financial advantage is lost. Physicians leading group visits must be trained and their first groups should be attended by an experienced mentor. A tendency exists to turn group visits into patient education classes, which is not their only purpose. Group visits are clearly not for everyone. Not all patients are interested in sharing their medical care and experiences in a group format. However, when offered, many patients appear to be willing to participate in group medical visits [8], making this form of alternative encounter a reasonable option for at least a segment of a practice's patient population.

The Improving Chronic Illness Care program of the MacColl Institute for Healthcare Innovation has developed an excellent group visit starter kit [9]. Portions of the starter kit are available in Appendix I.

VIRTUAL ENCOUNTERS

Group visits are one alternative to the one-on-one clinical encounter. At the other end of the spectrum lie virtual visits or encounters, a collection of alternative encounters strikingly different from the close-knit human interactions that characterize group visits. Virtual encounters consist of patient-clinician interactions that occur at a distance rather than as a face-to-face encounter.

Virtual encounters are a form of telemedicine. The Institute of Medicine has defined telemedicine as the use of electronic information and communications technologies to provide and support health care when distance separates the participants [10]. It includes such technologies such as telephones, faxes, two-way interactive video, digital imaging, health care monitoring devices, e-mail, and the Internet. The remaining sections of this chapter focus on two of these modalities of telemedicine: telephone care and e-mail/Internet communication.

Telephone Care

In adult medicine primary care, 25% of patient contacts are made via the telephone; in pediatrics, this proportion is even higher [11]. For brief exchanges of information between caregivers and patients, telephone care usually functions very well. However, the traditional use of telephone communication in primary care has some limitations. Telephone care for the most part happens on an impromptu basis, in response to an immediate patient care issue: concern about a new symptom, a request for a medication refill, a need to inform a patient about an abnormal test result [12]. Less often is telephone care a more proactive part of the clinician-patient interaction designed to substitute for face-to-face encounters.

Innovative approaches to telephone care include structured telephone care *appointments* and computer-assisted automated telephone care.

Telephone Appointments: The basic premise of telephone appointments is that a planned visit occurs over the telephone instead of in person. The telephone appointment is scheduled like a planned face-to-face visit, with a specific time booked on the clinician's schedule for the telephone visit. In an often-cited study published in 1992, Wasson and colleagues performed a randomized trial in Veterans' Administration (VA) clinics comparing two models of ambulatory care. One group of patients was randomized to a care model that required physicians to see patients less frequently for follow-up clinic visits but added scheduled phone calls between visits; the control group of patients received the usual approach to visit scheduling and no planned telephone appointments. The telephone-care patients had less medication use, fewer hospital days, and 28% lower expenditures compared with controls [13]. However, an attempt by Welch and colleagues to replicate Wasson's study several years later in different VA clinics found no benefit to scheduled phone calls [14]. Telephone appointments simply added to the number of patient encounters, rather than substituting for in-person visits, and patient outcomes were no better in the telephone appointment group.

Structured telephone appointments can involve members of the care team other than physicians. In a randomized controlled trial, patients with diabetes participating in telephonic case management had improved Hb A1c, blood pressure, and LDL-C levels compared with those receiving usual care [15]. A randomized controlled trial of patients with depression found that patients participating in eight sessions of telephone psychotherapy and care management had lower depression scores, and higher satisfaction with depression treatment than patients receiving usual depression treatment in primary care [16]. A study using pharmacists to make follow-up calls to patients soon after hospital discharge found that only 10% of patients receiving follow-up calls returned to the emergency department within 30 days, compared to 24% of patients in the group who were not called [17].

A major barrier to telephone appointments is lack of reimbursement by many payers, causing physicians paid fee-for-service to prefer a 15-minute visit (even if unnecessary) to a 5-minute phone call. Even under capitated or salaried payment, the business case for telephone visits is dependent on whether the phone visits substitute for in-person visits, or simply add to these visits. As the conflicting findings from the studies by Wasson and Welch described earlier suggest, the devil may lie in the details of how a telephone appointment program is implemented. Without a concerted effort to change established patterns and expectations for in-person visits, adding phone visits may simply supplement—rather than substitute for—face-to-face visits.

Computer-Assisted Automated Telephone Encounters: Nina Foner, a pediatrician, was amazed at how many hours her teenage son could spend in front of his computer screen doing his homework, researching assignments on the Internet, and instant messaging his friends. "Don't you believe in actually going to the library or talking to people any more?" she asked her son. "You're just old fashioned, Mom," her son replied. "Why don't you get with the new millennium!"

Dr. Foner decided to take her son's exhortations to heart. She and her practice partners decided that they weren't ready for a fully computerized practice, but they agreed that they could at least begin by automating their routine telephone services. Instead of having their medical assistants call families to remind them that their child was due for a checkup and immunization, they purchased a system to make computer-generated reminder calls. Once they became comfortable with that system, the vendor suggested that they add an option to allow families to select a prerecorded health education module as part of the automated phone care system. The automated call not only reminded the parents that their child was due for a visit, but also allowed the parents to punch in a number on the touch tone pad to select an age-appropriate health education message. Dr. Foner and her colleagues soon found that not only was their no-show rate falling, but also that families arrived at their visits more informed about child development issues.

Computer-assisted automated telephone encounters offer an even more radical departure from the traditional face-to-face encounter. This type of virtual visit entirely removes clinicians from direct participation in the encounter. Instead, the patient interacts by telephone with a computer programmed to produce voice messages and respond to information that a patient provides verbally or by touch tone. Piette has delineated the key functions of automated telephone care [17]. The most rudimentary function is performing administrative tasks. Many offices already use computer-generated telephone calls for one-way communication to remind patients about upcoming appointments. An extension of this administrative function involves reminders to patients about medication use or self-management action plans (see Chapter 5).

More sophisticated forms of automated telephone care add functions of patient monitoring and education—functions that are of particular value in the care of patients with chronic illness. Interactive voice response calls can monitor patients by prompting diabetic patients to report results of home blood glucose testing, or asthmatic patients to report peak flow measurements. These responses can be fed into a database and linked to an electronic medical record; the computer housing the database can also be programmed to alert a clinic nurse or case manager if patients report *outlier* values. Automated telephone calls may also incorporate electronic home monitoring devices that directly send information through the telephone line. For example, electronic scales for patients with heart failure can send data through a telephone modem; weight gains above a certain amount trigger an alert to the medical team that the patient may need an increased dose of diuretic medication.

Automated calls can also deliver patient education and counseling as part of a preventive or chronic care self-management program. Schillinger and colleagues designed an automated telephone service for patients with diabetes that, in addition to querying patients about self-management practices and blood glucose test results, also offers patients the option to listen to a prerecorded health education module [18]. These modules consist of vignettes about coping and self-management strategies told from a patient's point of view. This approach shares some of the goals of a group medical visit in its attempt to boost patients' self-efficacy through sharing of experiences and encouragement of patient self-activation.

Although there is not yet an extensive body of research evaluating automated telephone care, the existing evidence suggests that this type of virtual visit may be beneficial. Automated telephone reminders have been shown to increase vaccination rates among low-income patients, increase visit attendance rates for patients with tuberculosis, and assist patients in taking medications [17]. A great benefit of telephone care is the near-universality of telephones in people's homes (Table 7–1); this contrasts with the *digital divide* that limits the reach of e-mail and web-based clinical encounters (Table 7–2).

Automated telephone care systems for monitoring and self-management support have been found to improve clinical outcomes for patients with diabetes, asthma, heart failure, and chronic pain. Telephone care can also improve lifestyle behaviors and medication adherence [17]. One randomized trial of an automated telephone system for monitoring weights in patients with severe heart failure found a decrease in mortality

TABLE 7–1
Availability of telephone service among U.S. households

Households	With telephone	Without telephone
All households	98%	2%
White	98%	2%
African American	95%	5%
Hispanic	95%	5%
Over 65 years	99%	1%
Below poverty level	90%	10%

Source: Ref. 17.

TABLE 7-2	
Percentage households with Internet access, United States, October 2003	
Total population	58.7
White	65.1
African American	45.6
Hispanic	37.2
Employed	70.7
Not employed	42.8
Family income less than $15,000	31.2
Family income greater than $75,000	82.9
Less than high school education	15.5
College degree	84.9
Over 60 years, healthy	34.2
Over 60 years, multiple disabilities	8.3

Source: Ref. 22.

among the patients in the monitoring group [19]. No research has systematically evaluated the degree to which automated calls in practice function as substitutes or supplements for in-person primary care visits.

Automated telephone calls also have their drawbacks. The very notion of being called by a computer may seem fundamentally at odds with the primary care ethos of human interactions and personal relationships. However, research indicates that most patients actually find automated telephone care an acceptable and satisfying mode of communication, especially when it incorporates education and self-management counseling [20]. The versatility of this mode of communication may also be particularly valuable in caring for patient populations with low health literacy or limited English proficiency. Automated telephone messages can be tailored to specific literacy levels or be recorded in different languages [18].

The main limitation to automated telephone visits is the front-end investment needed to install a computerized call system and develop the interactive call content. Although the ongoing operating costs may be relatively low because of the automated nature of the communication, the initial investment may be considerable. The cost of implementing telephone care that provides education and self-management services for patients with specific chronic conditions requires a sufficiently large population of patients with the targeted conditions to justify the cost. For these reasons, automated telephone care systems have primarily gained a foothold in large health care organizations rather than small, independent physician offices.

E-mail and Internet

Compared with telephone care, e-mail and Internet's approaches to virtual visits have the potential to provide patients a more empowered role in their care. Many patients are frustrated with barriers to access to primary care face-to-face visits and would like to communicate with their physicians electronically [21]. In 2003, 59% of U.S. adults had access to the Internet and were using e-mail to communicate [22]. Around 2000, 90% of surveyed patients were interested in requesting medication refills, 87% in having nonurgent consultations, 84% in obtaining test results, and 78% in making appointments via e-mail [23].

E-mail and web-based communication are also appealing to primary care physicians and staff. As an asynchronous form of communication, the electronic medium helps avoid *telephone tag* and inconvenient interruptions, and provides better documentation since copies can be printed or attached to the electronic medical record. Electronic communication bypasses the problem of phone access faced by many primary care practices. Requests for lab results, prescription refills, monitoring of blood sugars, and nonurgent advice are ideal topics for electronic encounters [24].

Scherger writes: "A physician caring for about 2000 patients has about 40 patient interactions on any given day. Currently, 20–25 patients are seen each day in the office and the rest are handled by telephone. Many of these interactions could be handled by e-mail. The physician and other office staff would spend 1–2 hours a day on the computer, interacting with 20–30 patients. Our offices could be much quieter, with 30- to 60-minute appointments given to the 6–8 patients who really need to be seen" [25]. At one experimental primary care practice in Portland, Oregon, 80% of patient encounters take place by phone and e-mail, with only 20% as face-to-face visits [26].

In spite of these advantages to patients and providers, electronic communication has spread slowly in medical practice. In a 2000 survey of e-mail users, only 6% reported sending an e-mail message to their physician, although more than half wished to do so [27].

Physicians are worried that they will be inundated with volumes of inappropriate e-mail, which will consume time with no reimbursement.

Patients are concerned that the e-mail might not get to the right person or be answered promptly [21].

A serious problem with electronic virtual encounters is the *digital divide*—the lack of access to the Internet by people of lower income and less education (Table 7-2). In 2003, 65% of White households had Internet (including e-mail) connection, compared with 46% of African American and 37% of Latino households; 71% of households with employed members had Internet compared with 43% of unemployed households. The rate of increase in households connected to the Internet has slowed markedly in the past few years, suggesting that these disparities are slow to change [22]. Serious health care inequalities exist between the higher-income White population and vulnerable populations including people of low income, ethnic minorities, and non-English-speaking people; the digital divide could exacerbate these inequalities.

A randomized controlled trial of an e-mail system at two academic primary care centers revealed many positive aspects of e-mail use, but raised cautions about its capacity to improve primary care efficiency. About 100 physicians were randomized into two groups, one receiving e-mail directly from patients, the other having e-mail traffic triaged by a nurse who routed messages to the appropriate location. E-mail volume increased for the triage system, but not for the direct system, because the former was heavily promoted to patients of those physicians. In spite of greater e-mail volume, there was no significant difference in phone volume between the two groups of physicians. The triage physicians were more satisfied with e-mail. Patients using e-mail were younger and more educated than those who did not. Most patients liked e-mail for nonurgent problems, receiving test results, but preferred telephone for scheduling problems and discussing medication side effects. Over half of the patients surveyed said they preferred to speak with a *real person* and almost half felt that getting a response to e-mail took too long. Nearly half of the physicians felt that e-mails should be triaged by the clinic staff, but over half of the patients wanted e-mails to their physician seen only by the physician. This study suggests that electronic communication is acceptable to patients for a limited range of issues, that increasing electronic communication may not reduce telephone volume, and that visits and telephone encounters are the preferred modes of communication for many health matters [28].

Electronic communications between patients and providers must conform to the federal government's privacy standards for patient health information, mandated by the Health Insurance Portability and Accountability Act (HIPAA) of 1996. E-mail privacy is best protected by encrypting e-mail messages, adding another level of complexity to the use of e-mail. The American Medical Informatics Association (AMIA) and the American Medical Association have formulated guidelines for patient-physician e-mail communication; these include the caveat that urgent problems should not be communicated by e-mail. The AMIA guidelines recommend that physicians ask patients how they want to communicate with the practice and document in the chart which form of communication patients prefer for different purposes. The guidelines also recommend that physicians consider obtaining formal, informed consent for the use of e-mail [29].

Web messaging goes a step beyond basic e-mail, using a secure, web-based interface for electronic communication, which also actively sorts and routes electronic messages. A patient can log onto a secure Web site and send messages to the practice, indicating whether the communication is a request for medical consultation, obtaining test results, refilling a medication, or specialty referral. Communications can then be routed to different members of the practice based on the type of request (e.g., appointment requests to schedulers, consultation requests to an advice nurse or physician).

A university-run primary care practice owned by the University of California at Davis evaluated their implementation of a web-messaging system. The majority of patients found the system providing better access to their physician than the telephone. Most clinicians and staff were positive toward the system, though a number of clinic staff felt that it created more work. Physicians did not find the message volume to be onerous, and the face-to-face visit productivity of the practice as measured by RVUs (relative value units) actually increased after the system was introduced [23]. The authors speculated that the web-messaging system might have reduced the demand for visits, for medication refills and other simple needs, with the result that more in-person visits addressed higher-complexity health care needs. A study of Kaiser Permanente's use of web messaging found that the percentage of enrollees using electronic services to schedule appointments, request prescription refills, and ask medical questions increased markedly from 1999 to 2002. However, patients who were non-White and lived in low socioeconomic status neighborhoods were less likely to access e-health services, and this disparity worsened over time [30].

Betsy Powers loves being more in control of her and her family's health care, ever since her family's large multispecialty medical group implemented a web-based messaging and personal health record system. She uses her login ID and password to check her personalized Web site

*regularly. Just this week, the Web site wished her a happy fortieth birth-
day and alerted her that she might consider having a mammogram. Betsy
clicked on the link that took her to an interactive web page that assessed
her breast cancer risk and summarized the evidence on routine mammography. Seeing her relatively low-risk status, she decided to wait until age
50 to begin mammography screening. She switched login IDs and pass-
words and accessed the personalized page for her 12-year-old son, who
has epilepsy. There she found the results of her son's blood tests from the
previous day, showing the serum level of his anticonvulsant medications.
She saw that his levels were somewhat low, and consulting the medication
management plan her physician had provided her with, she noted that she
should give her son an extra dose of his medication for the following week
and schedule another blood test in a week. She was able to schedule the
blood test and follow-up physician visit over the web before she logged off.*

An even more ambitious extension of e-health technology includes the
functionality of web messaging with the additional capability of allowing
patients to access their electronic medical record directly over the Internet
and to make computer-facilitated health decisions. Under these types of
personal health record systems, patients can use a secure Web site to
obtain the results of diagnostic tests, review their list of prescribed medications, and access other aspects of their medical record. These Web sites
can also build in interactive technology that allows a patient to link to
information to assist in the interpretation of test results or provide additional interactive health education tailored to the patient's personal health
needs. One vision for these types of virtual visits sees highly individualized Internet technology replacing much of the content of routine medical
encounters. When a patient logs onto a Web site linked to an electronic
medical record, the computer would alert the patient of the age-
appropriate immunizations and cancer-screening tests that the patient had
not yet received. The patient could link to interactive educational modules,
about the risks and benefits of the recommended services, and then pro-
ceed to schedule appropriate services over the web. For a patient with
chronic illness, the computer could prompt the patient about routine interventions that were due, such as annual eye exams for diabetic patients.

Palo Alto Medical Foundation in California has been assessing its
development of a web-based patient portal through which patients can
view test results, access health information resources, request appointments, renew prescriptions, and communicate with their physicians
electronically. Monitoring surveys indicate that 90% of patients and
physicians are satisfied with the system, with patients reporting that the
system enhances their sense of partnership with the health care team [31].

The primary obstacle to taking full advantage of electronic technology for virtual visits is the capital investment and the lack of reimbursement for virtual visits that substitute for in-person visits [21]. One advantage that electronic virtual visits may have over telephone visits is that it is possible to program the computer for electronic visits to document and process a bill for the visit. Some payers have shown willingness to pilot payment schemes for electronic visits, provided there is adequate documentation for the visit [22].

CONCLUSION

The current health care system financially rewards primary care for the volume of face-to-face visits, and generally discourages the substitution of alternative forms of patient-clinician encounters. These financial disincentives may be weakening as more practices succeed in receiving reimbursement for group visits, and as payers are considering financial arrangements that would encourage phone and electronic communication. While proponents of alternative encounters persuasively argue that they will substitute for one-on-one face-to-face visits, thereby reducing the work of primary care practices, this increase in efficiency remains yet to be proven.

The sheer volume and pace of the 15-minute individual visit is the chief driver of the stress-producing hamster syndrome that creates early burnout for primary care clinicians. Alternative encounters that can rescue clinicians from the hamster treadmill are essential. Primary care practices will need to experiment with ingenious ways to reorganize their work flow such that group visits and virtual encounters reduce, rather than add to, the total volume of work.

REFERENCES

1. Scott JC, Conner DA, Venohr I, et al: Effectiveness of a group outpatient visit model for chronically ill older health maintenance organization members. J Am Geriatr Soc. 2004;52:1463–1470.
2. Noffsinger EB, Scott JC: Understanding today's group visit models. Group Pract J. 2000;49(2):48–58.
3. Beck A, Scott J, Williams P, et al: A randomized trial of group outpatient visits for chronically ill older HMO members. J Am Geriatr Soc. 1997;45:543–549.

4. Clancy DE, Cope DW, Magruder KM, et al: Evaluating concordance to American Diabetes Association standards of care for type 2 diabetes through group visits in an uninsured or inadequately insured patient population. Diabetes Care 2003;26:2032–2036.
5. Trento M, Passera P, Tomalino M, et al: Group visits improve metabolic control in type 2 diabetes. Diabetes Care 2001;24:995–1000.
6. Sadur CN, Moline N, Costa M, et al: Diabetes management in a health maintenance organization. Diabetes Care 1999;22:2011–2017.
7. Deakin T, McShane CE, Cade JE, et al: Group based training for self-management strategies in people with type 2 diabetes mellitus. Cochrane Database of Systematic Reviews 2005, Issue 2, CD003417.
8. Miller D, Zantop V, Hammer H, et al: Group medical visits for low-income women with chronic disease: a feasibility study. J Womens Health. 2004;13:217–225.
9. (*www.improvingchroniccare.org/improvement/docs/ startkit.doc*)
10. Field MJ (ed.), Institute of Medicine: *Telemedicine: A Guide to Assessing Telecommunications for Health Care.* Washington, DC, The National Academies Press, 1996.
11. Elnicki DM: Telephone medicine for internists. J Gen Intern Med. 2000;15:337–343.
12. Katz HP: *Telephone Medicine: Triage and Training for Primary Care.* Philadelphia, PA, F.A. Davis Company, 2001.
13. Wasson J, Gaudette C, Whaley F, et al: Telephone care as a substitute for routine clinic follow-up. JAMA. 1992;267:1788–1793.
14. Welch HG, Johnson DJ, Edson R: Telephone care as an adjunct to routine medical follow-up: a negative randomized trial. Eff Clin Pract. 2000;3:123–130.
15. Shea S, Weinstock RS, Starren J, et al: A randomized trial comparing telemedicine case management with usual care in older medically underserved patients with diabetes mellitus. J Am Med Inform Assoc. E-pub October 12, 2005.
16. Simon GE, Ludman EJ, Tutty S, et al: Telephone psychotherapy and telephone care management for primary care patients starting antidepressant treatment. JAMA. 2004;292:935–942.
17. Piette JD: *Using Telephone Support to Manage Chronic Disease.* Oakland, CA, California HealthCare Foundation, June 2005.
18. Handley MA, Hammer H, Schillinger D: Navigating the terrain between research and practice: a Collaborative Research Network (CRN) case study in diabetes research. J Am Board Fam Med. 2006;19:85–92.
19. Goldberg LR, Piette JD, Walsh MN, et al: Randomized trial of a daily electronic home monitoring system in patients with advanced heart failure. Am Heart J. 2003; 146:705–712.
20. Piette JD, Weinberger M, McPhee SJ: The effect of automated calls with telephone nurse follow-up on patient-centered outcomes of diabetes care. Med Care 2000;38:218–230.

21. Katz SJ, Moyer CA: The emerging role of online communication between patients and their providers. J Gen Intern Med. 2004;19:978–983.
22. *A Nation Online: Entering the Broadband Age.* U.S. Department of Commerce, September 2004. (*www.ntia.doc.gov/reports/anol/NationOnline-Broadband04.htm*)
23. Liederman EM, Morefield CS: Web messaging: a new tool for patient-physician communication. J Am Med Inform Assoc. 2003;10:260–270.
24. Bodenheimer T, Grumbach K: Electronic technology: A spark to revitalize primary care? JAMA. 2003;290:259–264.
25. Scherger JE: A new way of practicing. *Hippocrates.* August 2000, p. 8.
26. Kilo CM: Transforming care: medical practice design and information technology. Health Aff. 2005;24(5):1296–1301.
27. Moyer CA, Stern DT, Dobias KS, et al: Bridging the electronic divide. Am J Manag Care. 2002;8:427–433.
28. Katz SJ, Moyer CA, Cox DT, et al: Effect of a triage-based e-mail system on clinic resource use and patient and physician satisfaction in primary care. J Gen Intern Med. 2003;18:736–744.
29. Kane B, Sands DZ: Guidelines for the clinical use of electronic mail with patients. J Am Med Inform Assoc. 1998;5:104–111.
30. Hsu J, Huang J, Kinsman J, et al: Use of e-health services between 1999 and 2002: a growing digital divide. J Am Med Inform Assoc. 2005;12:164–171.
31. Tang PC, Lansky D: The missing link: bridging the patient-provider health information gap. Health Aff. 2005;24(5):1290–1295.

CHAPTER EIGHT

Computerizing the Primary Care Home

Dr. Dorothy Digital is a twenty-first century family physician. She carries a personal digital assistant (PDA) instead of a pager. She has no answering service; to communicate with her, patients e-mail her PDA, which sounds an alarm when a new e-mail arrives. Dr. Digital's face-to-face patient visits run from 11 a.m. to 1 p.m. and 3 p.m. to 5 p.m. For the remaining time she answers patients' e-mails (for which she is reimbursed by Medicare, Medicaid, and private insurers); analyzes home glucose results of her diabetic patients; titrates their medication doses on the Internet; examines her homebound, elderly congestive heart failure patients via her telemedicine hookup;, and beams prescription refills to the pharmacy from her PDA. Dr. Digital's office houses no books or patient charts. Evidence-based medical information is accessed instantaneously from Web sites, and all patient information is stored in the electronic medical record (EMR). Dr. Digital's medical assistant periodically sorts the patient registry and e-mails patients reminders to schedule a diabetic eye examination or come in for the third hepatitis B vaccination. Records from emergency department visits and hospitalizations appear in Dr. Digital's e-mail in-box and are transferred to the EMR. All patients carry electronic personal medical records with their problem and medication lists, allergies, recent laboratory data, and electrocardiographic tracing, data which is updated by synchronization with the EMR.

Advancements in technology have been a part of medicine from the time that an ancient healer first devised a better mortar and pestle for grinding medicinal herbs. Modern technological innovations stimulated specialization in medicine, with many specialties largely defined by mastery of technical procedures. Because technology has not defined primary care to the degree that it has other specialties, it is easy to overlook the ubiquitous and influential presence of technology in contemporary primary care offices. The stethoscope, the electrocardiogram machine, and even the telephone were once considered radical innovations; yet all became widely adopted as essential tools for primary care practice.

Innovation in computer technology is the most profound of recent technological advances. Electronic health care—e-health—is a development well suited to facilitating many key tasks of primary care. As Dr. Digital discovered, e-health is poised to become an essential element in the redesign of the primary care practice. Yet, it potentially threatens human relationships, fundamental to primary care, substituting impersonal exchanges across luminescent LCD screens for the face-to-face encounters and hands-on care that produce much of the therapeutic benefit and professional satisfaction of primary care practice. E-health could widen the disparities gap between patients with computer access and those without. Concerns abound that e-health, rather than making practice more efficient, may add new burdens, creating more work and additional expenses.

THE ROLES OF ELECTRONIC HEALTH CARE

E-health can be divided into several functional categories (Table 8–1): medical records, patient-clinician communication, clinician-clinician communication, and knowledge management [1].

TABLE 8–1
Functions served by e-health
Medical records
Communication
Patient-clinician
Clinician-clinician
Knowledge management
Information for clinicians
Information for patients

Medical Records

Medical records are a method for storing, organizing, and retrieving information about patients. For decades, medical records technology was markedly stagnant. Breakthroughs consisted of new systems of color-coded chart tags and rolling lateral file cabinets. A 1997 Institute of Medicine report begins: "In spite of more than 30 years of exploratory work and millions of dollars in research and implementation of computer systems in health care provider institutions, patient records today are still predominantly paper records" [2].

In 2002–2003, 17% of office-based primary care physicians used an EMR system [3]. In contrast, the great majority of primary care practices in the United Kingdom, Sweden, and other European nations are computerized [4]. In 2001, acknowledging the slow progress of medical record computerization, the Institute of Medicine recommended that public and private sectors of the health care economy "make a renewed national commitment to building an information infrastructure...[that will] lead to the elimination of most handwritten clinical data by the end of the decade" [5]. More rapid progress toward computerization is evident in hospital outpatient departments, integrated delivery systems, medical offices with 10 or more physicians, and practices with younger physicians [3].

In the paperless office, medical records would be entirely electronic, obviating the need for personnel to pull, file, and place reports in paper charts. The EMR system would interface laboratories, x-ray departments, hospitals, specialists, and pharmacies. The EMR system portals—whether computers, PDAs, voice recognition, or handwriting recognition devices— would be in every examination room and clinician's office; ideally, patients could view their computerized records along with their physicians.

EMR systems offer the promise of greater convenience, accessibility, integration, and accuracy of information about individual patients. Equally important, they can be a substrate for a population-based approach to medical practice that groups patients by diagnoses and clinical risk strata. Examples include chronic disease registries (see Chapter 4) and lists of patients appropriate for preventive services such as Papanicolaou tests or colon cancer screening. Early pioneers of population-based medicine devised systems of index cards with holes punched in the cards that allowed the physician to insert a rod to pull out cards for all patients with a particular diagnosis or characteristic—a technology with limited appeal to any but its true devotees. While many EMR systems lack these functionalities, they have the potential to offer a quantum leap in technology that facilitates sorting and retrieval of patient information to produce registries and reminder prompts.

Communication

Previous innovations in communications technology—the telephone and the pager—dramatically changed the accessibility of physicians to patients and colleagues. Computer technology offers additional novel means of communication.

Patient-Clinician: Many interactions—informing patients of test results, arranging specialty referrals, receiving data on home glucose levels and adjusting medication doses accordingly—can be handled by e-mail or web-based interactions, bypassing the frustrating telephone systems plaguing many medical facilities. These modalities are discussed in Chapter 7. Because some physicians are concerned that e-mail and web access will increase their workload, and because many insurers do not yet pay for electronic patient encounters, these communication modes are not yet prevalent in primary care. As one observer lamented, "many patients are beginning to use online communications and are dragging their doctors along" [6].

Clinician-Clinician: Electronic communication is gradually replacing the telephone and written correspondence for communications between primary care clinicians and specialists, as well as primary care practices and pharmacies. Specialty consultations can include an e-mail message with an electronic attachment of a patient's test results, a scanned photo of a skin lesion, or a digital radiograph.

The electronic prescription is a major breakthrough in physician-pharmacist communication. E-prescribing can be accomplished by using a PDA with software that produces lists of all products indicated for a particular diagnosis, provides proper dosages, flags drug interactions, determines whether the prescribed drug is on the patient's insurance or Medicare Part D formulary, and sends the prescription to the patient's pharmacy. A 2004 report found that 5–18% of physicians prescribe electronically [7].

Many hospitals have created portals, which allow staff physicians to access lab and x-ray results performed at the hospital for both inpatients and outpatients. Physicians without EMRs need to print the results from the computer terminal in their office; those with computerized records can ideally enter the results electronically into their EMR. In many cases, actual images—x-rays, MRI scans, ultrasounds, and coronary angiograms—can be transmitted. The most sophisticated portals allow primary care practices not only to receive but also to transmit information, including lab and x-ray requests, nursing, and medication orders.

An ultimate goal in provider-provider communication is the *Regional Health Information Organization (RHIO)*, which would link into a computerized network all hospitals, physicians, pharmacies, and other health-related institutions within a metropolitan area. Three communities—Indianapolis, Boston, and Santa Barbara—have become leaders in this effort. Most impressive is the work of the Regenstrief Institute in Indianapolis, which has developed a community-wide clinical data repository. Using patient privacy safeguards, this Indiana Network for Patient Care allows emergency department physicians to quickly access records, including for patients who usually receive care at different hospitals. Physician offices and physicians in hospitals are able to access the data from the repository [8].

Knowledge Management

Access to Information for Clinicians: On average, each ambulatory visit generates one clinical question that the physician is unable to answer [9]. Instantly accessible, up-to-date, evidence-based data should be a standard feature of any primary care practice, whether accessed on a computer or a PDA [10]. Medical information first became widely available via computer in 1971, when the National Library of Medicine began its MEDLINE system. Physicians conduct hundreds of millions of MEDLINE searches each year. As the Internet grew in the 1990s, nongovernmental medical sites developed, offering both commercial and noncommercial clinical information.

Using desktop computers or handheld PDAs, physicians can store or electronically access directories of pharmacies and specialists for each managed care panel, descriptions of medications including drug interactions, reference texts, practice guidelines, and evidence-based abstracts. Information can be downloaded to a PDA from a desktop computer or the Internet. These decision-support tools (one of the components of the Chronic Care Model discussed in Chapter 4) can also be embedded into EMR system software.

Access to Information for Patients: About 20% of adults in the United States use the Internet to access health information [11]. Holding contradictory views, 53% of users are distrustful of information they find on the Internet, but more than 70% report that the information influences health care decisions [12]. A growing number of patients bring online search results into their physicians' offices, expecting their physicians to interpret the information. As larger physician organizations initiate web-based patient portals (see Chapter 7), patients are likely to use health information from those portals.

TECHIES AND LUDDITES

Dr. Regina Webb returned from the Computers in Medicine conference enthused. "We need to get our e-mail and our Web site up and running, our EMR working, and let's save a few trees—get all this paper out of the office!" Her partner Dr. Rudolf Ludwig growled back, "You want to turn me into a secretary to type my chart notes into some stupid machine that breaks down every third day? You're going to spend megabucks for some system that will be obsolete in 2 years? And how do you expect to get laboratory results and discharge summaries from the hospital's ancient information system that doesn't talk to anyone else? Internet? Web? A patient came in here with a web printout demanding bone densitometry every year starting at age 40. The Web site was created by the company providing the densitometry. You go ahead and talk to your servers and browsers; I'll be talking to my patients."

If e-health has so much to offer, why isn't e-health technology more widely adopted in primary care practice? What are the barriers to e-health and how can these barriers be overcome (Table 8–2)?

E-Health Takes Too Much Time

One impediment to adoption is the fear that e-health technology will add to physicians' already demanding workload. Many physicians find that the time commitment involved in learning and using computers is too great, resulting in additional stress. Most studies have found that primary care physicians spend slightly more time working with an EMR system than with paper charts [13]. A pediatric computer algorithm increased compliance with management plans, but physicians found it too tedious to use during routine care [13]. A study of patient-physician e-mail communication at primary care sites concluded that the time physicians spent answering

TABLE 8–2
Some items to consider when computerizing primary care

- Does the electronic system save time or take more time?
- Is there an eventual financial benefit?
- Can the software connect with all other systems with which the practice needs to communicate?
- Is the software vendor reliable and stable over time?
- Are privacy concerns addressed?
- Do payers reimburse for services provided electronically?
- Does the computerized process enhance or hinder the clinician-patient relationship?
- Are workflows in the practice being redesigned to fit the electronic processes?
- How might computerization affect the practice staff and clinicians?
- What is the worst thing that can happen, and how can it be prevented?

patient e-mail requests was greater than the time saved on telephone calls and office visits. The authors predicted that as e-mail is used increasingly as a visit substitute, it would begin to reduce physician workload [14].

A hurdle for EMR systems is to overcome many physicians' resistance to typing. Voice-recognition software allows physicians to dictate into the EMR system, without typing or paying a transcriptionist, but these programs have thus far failed to perform with sufficient accuracy [15].

E-Health Is Too Expensive

Miller et al's 2005 in-depth study of 14 small primary care practices in 12 states found that initial costs to implement an EMR averaged $44,000 per full-time physician [16]. Ongoing costs averaged $8500 per physician per year, with a range of $6000 to $12,000. The EMR benefited the practices an average of $33,000 per physician per year. Most of the financial benefits came from the capacity to increase billing code levels and thereby generate higher revenues. In addition, practices were able to reduce personnel. The financial benefits derived from the EMR varied widely—between $6600 and $56,000 per physician per year—from one practice to another [16].

The sophistication of a practice in adopting and reaping savings from an EMR can be the difference between monetary gain and financial disaster. A paperless office can become a ghost town if the EMR system goes down, requiring budgets for uninterrupted power supplies, obsessive backup, and urgent technical assistance. A number of primary care practices have purchased EMR systems only to discontinue them [17].

Modifications to the full-scale EMR system are being developed to reduce the expense for small physician practices. A smaller system would computerize patient demographic data, problem and medication lists, and preventive care reminder prompts, but visit notes would be kept in paper charts [17]. Alternatively, the EMR system can computerize problem lists, medication lists, and chart notes but leave out reminder systems, chronic disease registries, and other decision-support tools. The partial EMR system can be upgraded later to add functionalities.

An alternative is the web-based EMR, in which the entire patient data warehouse is kept by a vendor and accessed via the Internet. This *application service provider* model burst on the health care scene in 1999. Rather than buying large new chunks of hardware, medical practices pay $100 to $600 per month per physician for the service. These products offer limited billing and scheduling systems or full EMR capability; they enable communication among physicians with different software packages. A risk of the web-based EMR is that all patient records are kept off-site [18].

Software Programs Come, Go, and May Not Talk to One Another

Can e-health seamlessly connect primary care physicians with specialists, hospitals, ancillary providers, and pharmacies? Currently, the everchanging array of vendors and software packages makes connectivity a problem. For example, prescriptions written on PDAs cannot always be transmitted electronically to pharmacies.

McDonald et al. make the analogy between the unconnected jumble of computer systems and a rain forest: "Within the rain forest, trees and other vegetation create a canopy, an interwoven system of plant life that provides a rich habitat...From the ground, the forest is a collection of individual trees. From the canopy, it is a seamless web" [19]. They argue that the Internet provides the opportunity for independent physician offices, pharmacies, laboratories, and hospitals to talk to one another, without each having the identical computer system. However, interoperability—the ability of software and hardware on different machines from different vendors to share data—has not yet overcome the syndrome of the Tower of Babel, the attempt to build a biblical structure which was abandoned when people spoke so many languages that they were unable to communicate.

Patient Privacy

To comply with the federal government's privacy standards for patient health information, mandated by the Health Insurance Portability and Accountability Act (HIPAA) of 1996, e-mail messages may be encrypted, adding another level of complexity to the use of e-mail. The American Medical Informatics Association and the American Medical Association have formulated guidelines for patient-physician e-mail communication; these include the caveat that urgent problems should not be communicated by e-mail, and they discuss e-mail–related liability and patient consent issues [20].

Lack of Reimbursement

A commonly expressed barrier to physicians' use of e-mail communication with patients is lack of reimbursement [20]. Although physicians paid by capitation or salary may face no disincentive to substitute virtual visits for in-person visits, the vast majority of practice revenue comes on a fee-for-service basis; substantial income is lost by reducing face-to-face patient encounters. While some insurers are paying fees for e-mail encounters, e-health use is unlikely to mushroom until the payment issue is resolved.

Patient-Clinician Relationship

A review of primary care computing suggests that both practitioners and patients are concerned about the possible negative impact of computers on the patient-physician relationship [13]. On a positive note, a study of physician-patient interactions before and after the introduction of exam room computers found that patient satisfaction increased with the use of the computer [21].

The Risks of Computerization

While many practices have successfully implemented EMRs, others have fallen on their faces. In one family medicine practice, little planning of the revised workflow took place resulting in less tracking of routine preventive and chronic care processes, greater interpersonal conflicts among practice staff, and an appointment scheduling nightmare [22]. Two of the practices studied by Miller et al. experienced severe billing problems that were at least partly EMR-related: "One had no billing or revenue for three months; another had no revenue for ten months (and nearly went bankrupt). A third had to redo its billing for the first six weeks after implementation and later endured a complete system crash that resulted in total loss of data and several weeks of providing care with no computer access or paper charts" [16].

In one internal medicine practice, the physicians encountered many challenges moving from paper to computer, including a lack of financial benefit, stressful redesign of the entire office workflow, a virus attack that crashed the system and disrupted telephone service, inadequate and expensive technical support, a feeling of incompetence by all practice staff as everything in the workday was new and mysterious, the ascension of a culture of blame as staff members and clinicians tried to pin fault on one another, and a temporary, dramatic increase in workload for physicians. Several patients asked such questions as "Doctor, do you find you are spending more time interacting with the computer than with your patients?" The physicians in the practice ultimately concluded that the EMR is an improvement over paper records, but the implementation process was a painful one [23].

Primary care practices may ask themselves, "Will we be one of the successes or one of the catastrophes?" Consulting with numerous colleagues who have been through the process is essential for practices planning EMR adoption.

THE BENEFITS OF COMPUTERIZATION

E-Prescribing

Quality improvement is associated with several functions performed by computerized clinical information systems. An in-hospital study found that computerized physician order entry reduced medication errors by 55% [24]. Nine of 15 studies on drug dosing systems—mostly within the hospital—demonstrated improved physician performance [25]. With the number of outpatient medication errors growing [26], it is likely that e-prescribing in the primary care setting can have salutary effects on patient safety [27].

Reminder Systems

Although clinical practice guidelines alone have not been shown to enhance quality, computerized reminders do improve physician compliance with practice guidelines [28]. Computerized reminder systems (see Chapter 4) improve clinical processes for a variety of conditions, including ordering tests to determine Hb A1c and lipid levels, conducting foot examinations, counseling smokers, increasing diabetic eye examinations, and others [29]; 14 of 19 studies of computerized reminder systems for preventive care showed improvement in processes of care; 19 of 26 studies examining computerized reminders or algorithms for a variety of medical conditions found a benefit [30]. Other reviews indicate that computerized reminders improve clinical processes for diabetes care, immunization, blood pressure screening, and Papanicolaou tests, although the improvements often fade if the reminders are stopped [13].

Physician Feedback

Compared with the laborious work of conducting chart audits, computerized clinical data systems can facilitate the provision of feedback to physicians on their clinical performance for preventive and chronic care (see Chapter 4). A Cochrane Review found that such feedback can improve both process and outcome measures in diabetes care [31]. A meta-analysis of interventions to improve physician performance in chronic care found that feedback to physicians had a modest but significant positive impact on clinical processes and outcomes [32].

Patient Self-Management of Chronic Illness

Studies are beginning to appear on the use of computers to assist patients in managing chronic conditions (see Chapter 5). One project to improve physical activity randomized diabetic patients to an Internet information-only program and an interactive program involving goal setting, reminders, and tracking of physical activity, web-based support from a personal coach, and web-based communication with other patients. In the intervention, those who logged onto the program frequently improved their amount of physical exercise, but as the weeks went by, this improvement waned [33].

Some vendors are hooking up patients to bathroom scales, blood pressure cuffs, and electrocardiogram machines, and providing home question-and-answer consoles to monitor symptoms; the electronically transmitted data are then analyzed by case managers. Claims abound that these programs save costs for hospital and emergency departments, but controlled trials are lacking [34].

A Caveat on Computerized Quality Enhancement

A recent study reveals the promise and limitations of electronic quality improvement. A controlled trial involving 13,000 adult diabetic patients used processes known to improve care such as computerized practice guidelines, diabetes registries for proactive population-based interventions, and performance feedback. The study found that most physicians did not use these computerized systems because they were too busy [35]. It confirmed that the electronic medium has potential to improve physicians' work lives and health care quality, but that this potential will not be actualized without carefully rethinking primary care workflow.

CONCLUSION

How can physicians in small practices begin to use electronic technologies in a manner that reenergizes rather than drains their professional lives? Instead of one giant step forward, computerization may occur in a staged manner with sequential addition of elements into an EMR system, beginning with patient demographics and problem and medication lists. Later, an EMR system may be programmed with reminder prompts for immunizations, preventive screening, and chronic care. Physicians can explore whether their local pharmacies are equipped to respond to electronic prescribing and determine which PDA software is compatible with their pharmacies' computer systems. An office e-mail policy can be developed after consultation with patients, colleagues, professional organizations such as the American Academy of Family Physicians, and the pharmacies, hospitals, and specialists with which the primary care practice interacts [36]. (Table 8–3)

Whichever innovations are chosen as a starting point, it is worthwhile to perform an analysis of the financial and workload implications of these

TABLE 8-3
Resources on computerizing primary care

American Academy of Family Physicians Center for Health Information Technology (*www.centerforhit.org*)

American College of Physicians Computers in Medicine (*www.acponline.org/computer/cim.htm*)

California HealthCare Foundation (*www.chcf.org*) click on iHealth and Technology

eHealth Initiative (*www.ehealthinitiative.org*)

Office of the National Coordinator for Health Information Technology (*www.hhs.gov/healthit/*)

changes. Electronic technology alters existing information and workflow patterns, and requires a conscious examination of practice procedures and office staff division of labor. If a practice institutes electronic reminder systems, medical assistants or nursing personnel can be trained to respond to computer prompts with minimal physician time commitment. If a practice begins using an e-mail system, procedures should be written for non-physician personnel to screen and triage e-mail communications, similar to procedures for handling telephone calls. Each electronic innovation should be tied to a change in office work patterns.

Electronic technology provides a powerful tool for generalists to keep abreast of relevant information from the expanding medical knowledge base and to serve their patients better. If computerization is performed in conjunction with simple alterations of workflow and division of labor, e-health may revitalize the primary care experience.

REFERENCES

1. Ebell MH, Frame P: What can technology do to, and for, family medicine? Fam Med. 2001;33:311–319.
2. Dick RS, Steen EB, Detmer DE (eds.): *Computer-Based Patient Record: An Essential Technology for Health Care.* Washington, DC, National Academy Press, 1997.
3. Burt CW, Sisk JE: Which physicians and practices are using electronic medical records? Health Aff. 2005;24(5):1334–1343.

4. Bates DW: Physicians and ambulatory electronic health records. Health Aff. 2005;24(5):1180–1189.
5. Institute of Medicine: *Crossing the Quality Chasm: A New Health System for the 21st Century*. Washington, DC, National Academy Press, 2001.
6. Kassirer JP: Patients, physicians, and the Internet. Health Aff. 2000;19(6): 115–123.
7. *Electronic Prescribing: Toward Maximum Value and Rapid Adoption*. Washington DC, eHealth Initiative, April 2004. (*www.ehealthinitiative.org*)
8. McDonald CJ, Overhage JM, Barnes M, et al: The Indiana Network for Patient Care: a working local health information infrastructure. Health Aff. 2005;24(5):1214–1220.
9. Bates DW, Ebell M, Gotlieb E, et al: A proposal for electronic medical records in U.S. primary care. J Am Med Inform Assoc. 2003;10:1–10.
10. Fischer S, Steward TE, Mehta S, et al: Handheld computing in medicine. J Am Med Inform Assoc. 2003;10:139–149.
11. Baker L, Wagner TH, Singer S, et al: Use of the Internet and e-mail for health care information. JAMA. 2003;289:2400–2406.
12. Brodie M, Flournoy RE, Altman DE, et al: Health information, the Internet, and the digital divide. Health Aff. 2000;19(6):255–265.
13. Mitchell E, Sullivan F: A descriptive feast but an evaluative famine. BMJ. 2001;322:279–282.
14. Katz SJ, Moyer CA, Cox DT, et al: Effect of a triage-based e-mail system on clinic resource use and patient and physician satisfaction in primary care: a randomized controlled trial. J Gen Intern Med. 2003;18:736–744.
15. Mohr DN, Turner DW, Pond GR, et al: Speech recognition as a transcription aid. J Am Med Inform Assoc. 2003;10:85–93.
16. Miller RH, West C, Brown TM, et al: The value of electronic health records in solo or small group practices. Health Aff. 2005;24(5): 1127–1137.
17. Chambliss ML, Rasco T, Clark RD, et al: The mini electronic medical record: a low-cost, low-risk partial solution. J Fam Pract. 2001;50: 1063–1065.
18. Bazzoli F: Is there an ASP in your future? Internet Health Care Magazine. July/August 2000:54–61.
19. McDonald CJ, Overhage JM, Dexter PR, et al: Canopy computing. JAMA. 1998;280:1325–1329.
20. Moyer CA, Stern DT, Katz SJ, et al: We got mail. Am J Manag Care. 1999;5:1513–1522.
21. Hsu J, Huang J, Fung V, et al: Health information technology and physician-patient interactions. J Am Med Inform Assoc. 2005;12:474–480.
22. Crosson JC, Stroebel C, Scott JG, et al: Implementing an electronic medical record in a family medicine practice. Ann Fam Med. 2005;3:307–311.
23. Baron RJ, Fabens EL, Schiffman M, et al: Electronic health records: Just around the corner? or over the cliff? Ann Intern Med. 2005;143:222–226.

24. Bates DW, Leape LL, Cullen DJ, et al: Effect of computerized physician order entry and a team intervention on prevention of serious medication errors. JAMA. 1998;280:1311–1316.
25. Hunt DL, Haynes B, Hanna SE, et al: Effects of computer-based clinical decision support systems on physician performance and patient outcomes. JAMA. 1998;280:1339–1346.
26. Phillips DP, Christenfeld N, Glynn LM: Increase in U.S. medication error deaths between 1983 and 1993. Lancet. 1998;351:643–644.
27. Schiff GD, Rucker TD: Computerized prescribing. JAMA. 1998;279: 1024–1029.
28. Solberg LI: Guideline implementation. Jt Comm J Qual Improv. 2000;26: 525–537.
29. Demakis JG, Beauchamp C, Cull WL, et al: Improving residents' compliance with standards of ambulatory care. JAMA. 2000;284:1411–1416.
30. Hunt DL, Haynes B, Hanna SE, et al: Effects of computer-based clinical decision support systems on physician performance and patient outcomes. JAMA. 1998;280:1339–1346.
31. Jamtvedt G, Young JM, Kristoffersen DT, et al: Audit and feedback: effects on professional practice and health care outcomes. Cochrane Database Syst Rev. 2006 (2): CD000259.
32. Weingarten SR, Henning JM, Badamgarav E, et al: Interventions used in disease management programs for patients with chronic illness–which ones work? BMJ. 2002;325:925–932.
33. McKay HG, King D, Eakin EG, et al: The diabetes network. Diabetes Care. 2001;24:1328–1334.
34. Celler BG, Lovell NH, Basilakis J: Using information technology to improve management of chronic disease. Med J Aust. 2003;179: 242–246.
35. Baker AM, Lafata JE, Ward RE, et al: A web-based diabetes care management support system. Jt Comm J Qual Improv. 2001;27:179–190.
36. MacDonald K, Metzger J: *Achieving Tangible IT Benefits in Small Physician Practices*. Oakland, CA, California HealthCare Foundation, 2002.

CHAPTER NINE

Health Care Teams in Primary Care

The notion of a health care team is as rarely challenged in principle as it is achieved in practice. Currently, a resurgence of interest in team-based care is evident. The Institute of Medicine has called for a *New Health System for the Twenty-First Century* with primary care teams playing a central role [1]. The quantum leap in the complexity of tasks prevents physicians alone from coping with the scope of practice. The imperative of cost containment leads provider organizations to favor lower-paid clinicians over physicians. The demand for quality encourages primary care to add caregivers with skills that physicians may not possess.

Will the primary care team come of age in the twenty-first century? This chapter begins by addressing the fundamental question: "What is a team?" Two practice organizations are described that highlight key characteristics of high-functioning teams. Research studies of teams in primary care elucidate the requirements of successful team building and also provide sobering evaluations of existing teams. The chapter concludes with some pointers on implementing a team structure in primary care practice.

GROUPS AND TEAMS

In health care settings, individuals from different disciplines come together to care for patients: the surgeon, nurse, and anesthesiologist in the

155

operating room; the oncologist, radiation therapist, and surgeon for patients with cancer; and the physician, nurse practitioner, medical assistant, and receptionist in the primary care office. These groupings conform to one definition of a patient care team as "a group of diverse clinicians who communicate with each other regularly about the care of a defined group of patients and participate in that care" [2].

But is a group of people who happen to be thrown together in a surgical suite or primary care office truly a team?

Dr. Mike Loner works in a private practice that includes a general internist and himself. He begins his 20-minute visit with Aaron Moore, a patient with hypertension, coronary heart disease, and chronic kidney disease, by thumbing through the chart to find the results from his most recent low-density lipoprotein cholesterol, creatinine, and prostate-specific antigen tests. The office has a medical records clerk never trained to perform these tasks. Dr. Loner then spends 5 minutes comparing the eight medication bottles brought by Mr. Moore with the chronic medication list in the chart, noting that Mr. Moore appears to be taking both 40-milligram and 20-milligram strength benazepril pills each day, instead of just the 40-milligram tablet that had been prescribed in the last visit with instructions to stop the 20-milligram pill. Reviewing the health maintenance form, he leaves the room to request a medical assistant to draw up pneumonia and influenza immunizations, finding the medical assistant sitting at her desk waiting for instructions about what to do next. Returning to the examination room, Dr. Loner learns that Mr. Moore has been unable to obtain an appointment with the urologist for a prostate biopsy; the doctor promises to arrange the appointment himself. As Mr. Moore leaves, Dr. Loner realizes that he did not need a medical degree to accomplish the tasks he performed during the medical visit.

Few people would argue that Dr. Loner, the medical records clerk, and the medical assistant—although working together to care for the same patients—truly function as a team.

A consideration of teams evokes two questions: "Who should be the players on the team?" and "How can the players act as a team rather than as a collection of individuals?" A familiar team is a football squad. Football teams need the right mix of players. A 22-member team with 11 quarterbacks and 11 defensive linebackers would win few games. Similarly, a primary care practice with three physicians and no receptionist, medical assistant, or billing clerk is seldom a winning combination. Even with the right mix of players, a football team with no plays, no practice sessions, and no game plan would be unlikely to land in the Super Bowl. In fact, such a *team* is not truly a team but simply a group of individuals. Even though groups of health care personnel thrown together in an office, clinic, or hospital floor are generally called teams, they need to earn true team status by demonstrating teamwork [3].

A simple definition of team may help to distinguish unstructured groups versus organized teams: "A team is a group with a specific task or tasks, the accomplishment of which requires the interdependent and collaborative efforts of its members" [4]. The football example clarifies the difference between a group and a team:

> It is naive to bring together a highly diverse group of people and expect that, by calling them a team, they will in fact behave as a team. It is ironic indeed to realize that a football team spends 40 hours a week practicing teamwork for the two hours on Sunday afternoon when their teamwork really counts. Teams in organizations seldom spend two hours per year practicing when their ability to function as a team counts 40 hours per week [4].

A BRIEF HISTORY OF PRIMARY CARE TEAMS IN THE UNITED STATES

The general practitioner of the early twentieth century was a lone ranger. Black bag in hand, he treated and comforted patients, often in their homes. As office practice emerged, the first primary care team was husband and wife, the wife serving as receptionist, billing clerk, and bookkeeper. As practice became more complex, nonphysician tasks became further subdivided into receptionist, medical assistant, and billing clerk, a pattern found in the myriad of small practices dotting the United States.

In 1915, teams of physicians, health educators, and social workers were created at Massachusetts General Hospital's outpatient department. Primary care team models were developed at New York's Montefiore Hospital in 1948 and at Yale in 1951 [4]. The Neighborhood Health Center program of the 1960s developed primary care teams in some early health centers [5, 6]. Larger group practices also incorporated a diverse complement of health professionals into teams.

Despite these efforts, primary care teams did not become the dominant paradigm. One obstacle was the "overwhelming barriers of disciplinary territoriality and systems inertia" [7]. Payment systems failed to reimburse work performed by nonphysician professional members of the team, undermining the financial viability of teams. Perhaps most critical was the failure to articulate the objectives of a team model and to provide evidence on the advantages of team models for achieving these objectives. The *team meeting*—lengthy sessions in which each team member offered his or her perspective on a patient and family—became emblematic of these failures. Dr. Ron Goldschmidt, a physician veteran of the 1970s team practice, writes:

> Because our goals were so lofty, we needed to spend enormous amounts of time together to explore all the intricacies and nuances of comprehensive health care...The central organizing event was the pre-clinic meeting, usually held at one of a number of local restaurants. Quite regularly, critical decisions were made at this time. The most memorable of these was restaurant selection for the next week. The patients/families? No one really knows how it was for them.

At the start of the twenty-first century, do well-functioning primary care teams exist in the United States? Two case studies highlight organizations striving toward high-performing teams. One setting is a small private office, the other a large group practice.

TWO CONTEMPORARY PRIMARY CARE TEAMS

Dr. Charles Burger

Charles Burger is a private practitioner in Bangor, Maine. From a distance, this remarkable primary care practice resembles thousands of physician offices throughout the country. Upon entering the office door, it is clear that—within a traditional practice setting—Dr. Burger has created a smoothly functioning primary care team. The entire office functions as one team—two physicians and two nurse practitioners are the clinicians, complemented by medical assistants, greeters, receptionists, and schedulers. The practice is financially stable and busy, with each clinician seeing 23–30 patients per day. The following fictional case typifies how the team model works:

Ms. Carlotta Belli called Dr. Burger's office complaining of recurrent abdominal discomfort after eating. The receptionist consulted her computerized triage protocol and told Ms. Belli to come the same day. When she arrived, the greeter, already aware of the patient's problem, gave her a medical history questionnaire specifically related to abdominal pain, which Ms. Belli filled out in the waiting room. Ms. Belli met with the medical assistant who checked her vital signs and quickly entered her questionnaire responses into the computer. Ms. Belli then saw the physician, who reviewed the history, performed a relevant physical examination, and consulted a diagnostic software program. Discussing the options with Ms. Belli, the physician and patient decided on a diagnostic and treatment plan. Ms. Belli then met with the scheduler, who arranged laboratory and ultrasound studies.

Dr. Burger's staff members were all trained at a 15-week course in quality management at a nearby college. Greeters, receptionists, and schedulers (who are cross-trained) also received 6 weeks of in-office training.

All clinical processes in Dr. Burger's office are guided by a system. The practice has adopted advanced access scheduling, offering patients same-day appointments. For years, the office has tracked demand and can predict how each day will unfold. On Mondays, heavy with telephone calls, more staff act as receptionists and few scheduled appointments are made.

Although in most offices, receptionists are not trained properly to triage patients into emergency, urgent, and routine categories, Dr. Burger designed a triage system that receptionists consult on every telephone call. When Ms. Belli called with abdominal complaints, the receptionist pulled up the gastrointestinal screen on the triage protocol, which prompted a series of questions including pain severity and presence of vomiting, diarrhea, black and/or bloody stools, or fever. In the case of positive answers, the protocol tells the receptionist to send Ms. Belli to the emergency department. For milder symptoms, an appointment is made, perhaps with previsit laboratory studies. The interaction is routed to Ms. Belli's medical record and a clinician's e-mail in-box.

Most communication is routinized by the office's clinical systems. Team members do not attend endless meetings, incoming calls are routed to the e-mail in-box of the appropriate team member, urgent messages are delivered in person, and diagnostic studies go to the appropriate e-mail in-box and the medical record. The well-trained medical assistants order clinical preventive studies based on the patient's age and sex. Clinic goals and performance measures are communicated to all the staff by posters prominently displayed in the office.

Kaiser Permanente in Georgia

At the opposite end of the primary care spectrum is Kaiser Permanente's large delivery system. In 1997, Kaiser Permanente's Georgia region (KP/Georgia) developed primary care teams with several goals: increased patient satisfaction, improved Health Plan Employer Data and Information Set scores, and lowered costs.

This group practice model currently consists of 9 primary care offices with 25 teams. Each team has 3–5 clinicians (physicians, nurse practitioners, or physician assistants), 2 registered nurses, 1–2 receptionists or clerks, and 6–7 licensed practical nurses or medical assistants, providing care to a panel of 8000–15,000 patients. Prior to the rollout of the team structure, clinicians and staff received training in team-oriented care.

Patients view their clinician, not the team, as their primary caregiver, but are aware that a nonphysician clinician may provide care for acute problems or if the physician is not available. Eighty-five percent of visits are handled by a clinician on the patient's team.

Kaiser Permanente's Georgia team, like Charles Burger's practice, has well-defined systems and protocols for all clinical processes including triaging telephone calls, reviewing and informing patients of laboratory and x-ray results, making referrals, and renewing prescriptions. One registered nurse is the advice nurse answering patient questions and triaging patients who telephone or drop-in. The other registered nurse is the team co-leader, working with the physician co-leader to solve day-to-day problems, to ensure that clinical systems are functioning well and to supervise team members.

Each team receives a budget based on the number of patients on the team's panel with risk adjustment according to age and disease severity. Initially given limited decision-making autonomy, teams demonstrating effective self-management are allowed flexibility in staffing mix and division of labor. Teams can decide if they want more physicians, nonphysician clinicians, or support staff in their personnel mix. Some teams delegate chronic care management functions to licensed practical nurses and medical assistants; others are less successful in this redesign. Each team decides how chronic disease registries are used to improve its panel's outcome measures. Some use the registries extensively, others minimally.

Each team receives a quarterly report on team functioning, patient satisfaction, staff satisfaction, and clinical quality measures, enabling KP/Georgia's central leadership to assess each team's functioning and allowing each team to compare itself with other teams.

BUILDING TEAMS

What are the features that distinguish the teams of Charles Burger and KP/Georgia from the dysfunctional working group of the fictional Dr. Loner? The conceptual work of several scholars has highlighted five key elements of team building: clear goals with measurable outcomes, clinical and administrative systems, division of labor, training, and communication [3, 7–9]. Both Dr. Burger's practice and the KP/Georgia teams exemplify these elements. Both of these practices have concrete goals and measure their performance in reaching these goals, for example, patient satisfaction, good clinical outcomes, and in the case of KP/Georgia, cost reduction. Both of these institutions have established detailed systems to accomplish the tasks that all primary care practices must fulfill. They have constructed a division of labor so that each team member knows, and is well trained to accomplish, the role he or she must play in performing each task. Dr. Burger's practice illustrates a creative approach to division of labor by devising nontraditional positions, such as the *greeter*, and by delegating to receptionists and medical assistants some tasks that are typically performed by clinicians. Practice systems, division of labor, and training are missing elements in the fictional practice of Dr. Loner. While Dr. Burger's practice makes a substantial investment in staff training, Dr. Loner—like many primary care practices— puts new employees to work after a scant 2-hour orientation. In the practices of both Dr. Burger and KP/Georgia, communication is accomplished via systems and protocols and by face-to-face, minute-to-minute conversations rather than by lengthy meetings (Table 9–1).

RESEARCH STUDIES ON PRIMARY CARE TEAMS

No one disputes the broad statement that health care is a team sport. But does a body of evidence tell us how to organize a successful team? Does a literature review demonstrate that teams in primary care can improve patient outcomes and create a more satisfying work environment? How many caregivers should be on a primary care team, and who should those people be? When a team structure is implemented in a primary care

---

TABLE 9–1

Key elements of team building

1. Defined Goals

   Overall organizational mission statement

   Examples:

   > Improvement of patient's health
   > Reduction in barriers to access to care
   > Improvement in practice's financial performance
   > Physician and staff satisfaction

   Specific, measurable operational objectives

   Examples:

   > At least 80% of diabetic patients will have hemoglobin A1c lower than 8
   > Ninety percent of people calling for a nonurgent appointment will receive the appointment within one week
   > Practice will achieve a targeted level of practice revenue
   > Each team member will achieve an explicitly identified goal for personal, professional development

2. Systems

   Clinical systems

   Examples:

   > Procedures for providing prescription refills
   > Procedures for informing patients of laboratory results

   Administrative systems

   Examples:

   > Procedures for making patient appointments
   > Policies on how decisions are made in the medical practice

3. Division of labor

   Definition of tasks

   Assignment of roles (Determining which people on the team perform which tasks within the clinical and administrative systems of the medical practice)

4. Training

   Training for the functions that each team member routinely performs

   Cross-training to substitute other roles in cases of absences, vacations, or periodic heavy demands on one part of the team

---

> **TABLE 9-1**
>
> **Key elements of team building (*Continued*)**
>
> 5. Communication
>
>   **Communication structures**
>
>   Examples:
>
>   Routine communication through paper and electronic information flow
>   Minute-to-minute communication through brief, verbal interactions among team members
>   Team meetings
>
>   **Communication processes**
>
>   Examples:
>
>   Giving feedback
>   Conflict resolution

practice, what actually happens? A detailed literature review addressing these questions is presented in Appendix O, examining the research on: (1) factors associated with well-functioning teams, (2) the association between teamwork and practice outcomes, and (3) the effects of different team compositions in primary care on patient outcomes. We briefly summarize the findings from this literature review here.

Factors Associated with Well-Functioning Teams

Studies on primary care teams serve as reminders that team-based care is an innovation requiring considerable doses of organizational expertise and human cooperation. In the words of one group of researchers, "Conflict is a natural and inevitable development of interdisciplinary team life" [10]. The organization within which the team functions—whether a small practice, in which the team is the entire organization, or a large institution with several or many teams—can create the conditions for a successful team or can undermine the efforts of the team. The team can be dysfunctional, leading to low morale, high turnover, and poorer patient outcomes or it can be cohesive and high performing, learning from the research on and experience of actual teams.

A team is only as good as the individuals in it. Some teams have highly competent and collaborative members, while others do not. Assuming a reasonable level of competence and cooperativeness of team members, some teams do perform as an organism that is greater than the sum of its parts, while other teams do not. Factors associated with better performance include good leadership, a clear division of labor, training of team members in their personal roles and in team functioning, and team-supporting policies of the organization within which the team is working. A favorable organizational climate (of the larger organization) appears to be associated with improved team cohesion. Considerable and ongoing investment is required to create and sustain team cohesion. This investment includes the training of team members in team functioning, creation of protocols that define who on the team does which tasks, adoption of team rules including decision making and communication, and granting of some protected, non–patient–care (i.e., noneconomically productive) time for team meetings. No formal economic study has been published examining whether the downtime, set aside for team meetings in primary care, may actually produce some offsetting financial benefit through improved overall team productivity or decreased staff absenteeism and turnover.

Teamwork and Practice Outcomes

The few studies that have investigated team cohesion and related measures of teamwork and their association with operational effectiveness suggest that greater team cohesion is associated with improved clinical outcomes of the team's patients. For example, a study of general practices in England found that performance in diabetes care, overall patient satisfaction, continuity of care, and access to care were significantly higher in practices with higher scores on assessments of team climate. Clinical quality for asthma, coronary heart disease, and preventive services were not significantly associated with team climate [11]. Researchers have studied the KP/Georgia teams described earlier in this chapter; initial findings suggest that teams with higher "collaborative clinical culture" scores have superior patient outcomes, including better patient satisfaction and better control of diabetes and hyperlipidemia [12].

Who Should Be the Players on the Team?

One motivation for adding team members is to conserve expensive physician labor through substitution of lower-cost personnel for physician effort.

Most formal research on substitution in primary care has examined the role of nonphysician clinicians, that is, nurse practitioners and physician assistants. Two recent meta-analyses provide evidence that nurse practitioners can deliver care of equivalent quality to that delivered by primary care physicians [13, 14], with the caveat that most studies reviewed included small numbers of clinicians and few examined long-term outcomes for patients with chronic illness or complex conditions.

Research is inconclusive about whether substitution of personnel with lower salaries in primary care always translates into lower cost per visit. Although several studies indicate that the use of nonphysician clinicians can reduce costs in primary care practices [15, 16], some of these studies have been criticized for not accounting fully for nonphysician clinicians seeing fewer patients per hour and working fewer hours per week than primary care physicians [17]. A recent study of primary care teams in Kaiser Permanente's Georgia region, carefully accounting for visit productivity and work effort, concluded that teams that made greater use of nurse practitioners and physician assistants relative to physicians had lower overall team labor costs per visit [18].

Configuring team personnel is not just a matter of substitution for economic benefit. Another objective is enhancement of clinical performance. Team members may contribute unique talents that enhance the skill mix of the practice. Numerous studies suggest that multidisciplinary clinical teams produce clinical outcomes superior to those achieved by usual care arrangements, with many of these studies evaluating the addition of nurses, social workers, psychologists, and clinical pharmacists to teams [2]. One limitation these studies have is that extra personnel conveys an advantage, and it may be unclear whether it was better teamwork or a larger team that produced the benefit.

A recent randomized trial in the Netherlands has elucidated the substitution versus enhancement issue. Several general practices added nurse practitioners to their teams to focus on the care of patients with chronic conditions, with the expectation that physicians would delegate many chronic care tasks to the nurse practitioners. Although access to care for the targeted patients improved in the teams with nurse practitioners, the general practitioners reported no decrease in their practice workload overall or for patients with chronic conditions. In other words, nurse practitioners enhanced services but did not substitute for physicians. The authors concluded, "Gains for the efficiency of services can be achieved only if general practitioners give up providing the types of care they have delegated to nurses and instead invest their time in activities that only doctors can perform" [19].

THE PROBLEMS WITH TEAMS

If teams are such a good idea, why aren't they more prevalent? As the above research demonstrates, teams have some inherent drawbacks related to their added organizational complexity. As team size increases, the transaction costs of interpersonal communication increase exponentially and may overtake the benefits of teamwork [20]. Team size may have a U-shaped relation to teamwork; too few or too many team members reduce effectiveness [8]. One study suggests that 6 team members is the optimal size; teams with greater than 12 members are too large [21]. Teams also require dealing with the challenges of human relationships and personalities [22]. While some team members may shine as initiators, clarifiers, or encouragers, others may play negative roles as dominators, blockers, evaders, and recognition seekers [3].

Despite evidence that teams may enhance clinical performance, delegating tasks to other team members may erode work satisfaction for the generalist physician attracted by the idea of personally delivering comprehensive care. The undifferentiated and varied nature of clinical problems in primary care makes team building especially challenging. A single-specialty practice will find it relatively easy to delineate tasks and define roles, compared with a primary care practice facing a more diffuse array of clinical tasks.

It is difficult to meld the reality that some team members are more expert than others, requiring hierarchy, with the importance of all members fully participating in team functioning. Similarly, collaborative decision making is a challenge when physicians are used to (and sometimes should be) giving clinical orders to other caregivers [23].

Finally, financial incentives matter. Economic disincentives are prominent under current fee-for-service payment policies; an office visit with a physician or nurse practitioner, but not with a medical assistant, is billable, negating the economic benefit of the practice of substitution.

INTRODUCING TEAMS INTO PRIMARY CARE

Organizing primary care practices into teams is not a simple undertaking. But one overriding reality places research on teams into bold perspective—primary care has no choice. The current structure of most practices—with no teams or with loosely structured teams—is not working. As described in

Chapter 1, physicians lack the time to perform all the functions expected of primary care. Physicians need to delegate; other caregivers need to assume partial responsibility for the care of the practice's patients. That inevitable transformation equals a team.

Teams are a necessary substrate upon which other innovations— the Chronic Care Model, advanced access, group visits, and electronic encounters—can be catalyzed. The question is less "Should there be teams?" and more "How can teams set and achieve goals—both lofty and realistic— for their members and their patients?"

Primary care practices can take small, initial steps toward creating more effective teamwork. Building a cohesive primary care team begins with an assessment of one's own working group, using key elements of team building (Table 9–1) as a guide. One place to begin is a tool provided in Appendix C, a brief questionnaire for staff and clinicians that assesses team members' perceptions of their work processes. Does the practice have clearly articulated clinical, business, and work environment goals with measurable outcomes to assess improvement? One English general practice successfully pioneered a process of engaging clinicians and staff to agree on practice goals [24]. Once the goals are formulated, does the practice have the best mix of personnel to meet the goals?

Do detailed systems exist to routinize practice tasks, for example, how patient telephone calls are triaged, how laboratory and x-ray results (normal or abnormal) are communicated to patients, and how refills for different categories of prescriptions are handled? Does each team member have clearly defined tasks within these systems and is each well trained to perform those tasks? Appendices B, C, D, E, and H provide tools for assessing basic clinical and administrative systems that operate in a primary care practice.

Could nonphysician personnel substitute for physicians in performing some tasks, thereby decompressing physician workload? Practices frequently underuse the capabilities of receptionists and medical assistants. In the vignette about Dr. Loner, the medical records clerk could have been trained to maintain a flow sheet with patient laboratory data and the medical assistant could have been taught how to make specialty appointments for elderly patients unable to navigate the health system. A medical assistant could have been trained in comparing the patient's medication list with the pills the patient was actually taking, saving Dr. Loner 5 minutes of the medical visit. Low-cost investment in staff training—either on-the-job or in local community colleges—can unleash the full potential of team members. The training does require physicians to spend time up front, an investment that should save physicians like Dr. Loner substantial time in the long run.

Barriers to team development are considerable. A predator of the primary care team is the hamster [25]. Hamster health care—the rapidly revolving treadmill upon which so many clinicians find themselves—creates a state of mental exhaustion that frustrates attempts at planning and cooperation. Though a well-functioning team with a clear division of labor might relieve physicians of some of their workload, finding the time to participate in team development is difficult for physicians. Whether or not a primary care practice chooses to focus on team development as a major innovation, many practices may benefit by introducing or improving one or more components of high-performing teams—clear goals with measurable outcomes, defined tasks and roles, clinical and administrative systems with a clear division of labor, and effective communication. Making time to step off the treadmill to invest in team planning may yield long-term benefits in the form of an improved work environment.

REFERENCES

1. Institute of Medicine: *Crossing the Quality Chasm: A New Health System for the 21st Century*. Washington, DC, National Academy Press, 2001.
2. Wagner EH: The role of patient care teams in chronic disease management. BMJ. 2000;320:569–572.
3. Fried BJ, Rundall TG, Topping S: Groups and teams in health services organizations. In: Shortell SM, Kaluzny AD, eds: *Health Care Management*. Albany, NY, Delmar Thomson Learning, 2000.
4. Wise H, Beckhard R, Rubin I, et al: *Making Health Teams Work*. Cambridge, MA, Ballinger Publishing Co, 1974.
5. Lashof JD: The Health Care Team in the Mile Square Area, Chicago, IL Bull N Y Acad Med. 1968;44:1363–1369.
6. Wise H: The primary care team. Arch Intern Med. 1972;130:438–444.
7. Baldwin DC: *The Role of Interdisciplinary Education and Teamwork in Primary Care and Health Care Reform*. Washington, DC, Health Resources and Services Administration, Department of Health and Human Services, 1994.
8. Cohen SG, Bailey DE: What makes teams work: group effectiveness research from the shop floor to the executive suite. J Manag. 1997;23:239–290.
9. Rubin IM, Beckhard R: Factors influencing the effectiveness of health teams. Milbank Mem Fund Q. 1972;50:317–335.
10. Sands RG, Stafford J, McClelland M: 'I beg to differ': conflict in the interdisciplinary team. Soc Work Health Care. 1990;14:55–72.
11. Campbell SM, Hann M, Hacker J, et al: Identifying predictors of high quality care in English general practice: observational study. BMJ. 2001;323:1–6.

12. Roblin DW, Kaplan SH, Greenfield S, et al: Collaborative Clinical Culture and Primary Care Outcomes. Washington, DC, program and abstracts of the annual meeting of the Academy for Health Services Research and Quality, June 23–25, 2002.
13. Brown SA, Grimes DE: A meta-analysis of nurse practitioners and nurse midwives in primary care. Nurs Res. 1995;44:332–339.
14. Horrocks S, Anderson E, Salisbury C: Systematic review of whether nurse practitioners working in primary care can provide equivalent care to doctors. BMJ. 2002;324:819–823.
15. Grzybicki DM, Sullivan PJ, Oppy JM, et al: The economic benefit for family/ general practices employing physician assistants. Am J Manag Care. 2002;8:613–620.
16. Venning P, Durie A, Roland M, et al: Randomized controlled trial comparing cost effectiveness of general practitioners and nurse practitioners in primary care. BMJ. 2000;320:1048–1053.
17. DeAngelis CD: Nurse practitioner redux. JAMA. 1994;271:868–871.
18. Roblin DW, Howard DH, Becker ER, et al: Use of midlevel practitioners to achieve labor cost savings in the primary care practice of an MCO. Health Serv Res. 2004;39:607–626.
19. Laurant M, Hermens R, Braspenning J, et al: Nurse practitioners do not reduce the workload of GPs; a randomized controlled trial. BMJ. 2004;328:927–930.
20. Barr DA: The effects of organizational structure on primary care outcomes under managed care. Ann Intern Med. 1995;122:353–359.
21. Starfield B: *Primary Care: Balancing Health Needs, Services and Technology*. New York, Oxford University Press, 1998.
22. Lencioni P: *The Five Dysfunctions of a Team*. San Francisco, CA, Jossey-Bass, 2002.
23. Feiger SM, Schmitt MH: Collegiality in interdisciplinary health teams: its measurement and its effects. Soc Sci Med. 1979;13:217–229.
24. Adelaide Medical Centre Primary Health Care Team: A primary health care team manifesto. Br J Gen Pract. 1991;41:31–33.
25. Morrison I, Smith R: Hamster health care: time to stop running faster and redesign health care. BMJ. 2000;321:1541–1542.

CHAPTER TEN

Diagnosing and Treating the Primary Care Practice

Dr. Aaron Best was tired. He had seen 26 patients, it was 7 P.M., and a stack of phone messages, laboratory test results, and charts cluttered his desk. He had been off call the previous weekend, it was Monday, and he was already stressed out. The day hadn't gone well. The schedule had been full when he arrived in the morning and a 9 A.M. drop-in patient with tarry stools and a hematocrit of 23 had pushed everything back an hour. The exam rooms weren't stocked properly and Dr. Best was constantly running out to get referral forms, speculums, and patient education materials. Phone interruptions seemed incessant. There was no textbook or Internet access to help him figure out what to do with a patient just discovered to have an adrenal incidentaloma. One of Dr. Best's favorite patients informed him that she was changing to another physician because Dr. Best's practice was just too chaotic. The medical assistant announced that she was filing for workers' compensation for carpal tunnel syndrome. Dr. Best had been doing exactly what he had been trained to do—cope with all the things that get in the way of good care for his patients—and he was exhausted.

Chapter 1 reviewed a number of problems facing patients, clinicians, and nonprofessional caregivers in primary care practices. These problems include patient delays in accessing timely appointments, inadequate time to satisfy patient needs and desires in the brief office visit, high levels of clinician stress, and resultant deficiencies in chronic and preventive care.

While primary care overall confronts these problems and more, each particular primary care practice experiences these problems in its own distinct way. To solve its particular problems, a practice must first make a diagnosis of what those problems are, prioritize which are the most important, and then figure out solutions. In other words, medical practices need to diagnose and treat themselves.

A group of clinicians, researchers, and quality improvement experts at Dartmouth Medical School's Center for the Evaluative Clinical Sciences has developed a superb framework—called *microsystem analysis*—for diagnosing, prioritizing, and treating problems in medical practices. This chapter describes microsystem analysis and explores how it can be used to improve primary care.

WHAT IS A MICROSYSTEM?

The primary care practice is situated within a macrosystem, consisting of the population living in its vicinity and a multiplicity of health care institutions: Medicare, Medicaid, private health insurance plans, hospitals, specialists, ancillary services, pharmacies, home health agencies, and more.

A microsystem is the "local milieu in which patients, providers, support staff, information, and processes converge for the purpose of providing care to meet health needs" [1]. A primary care practice and its patients are a microsystem. Similarly, a specialty clinic with its patients or a hospice with its patients is a microsystem. Different microsystems interact with one another.

Many problems within the primary care home are exacerbated by negative influences emanating from the macrosystem, such as inadequate reimbursement or administrative hassles imposed by health plans. But other problems are rooted within the microsystem itself. It is those problems— the internal rather than the external factors—that microsystem analysis can help solve. Are the external influences important? Absolutely. However, improvement often starts from within the practice, in areas that can be controlled by the practice.

Multiple levels of health care are at work for any given patient in any particular place (Figure 10–1). The self-care level involves the patient and a source of information; the individual patient–individual caregiver interacting during the medical visit is the level for which physicians are trained; the clinical microsystem is the level at which most caregivers work—the small group

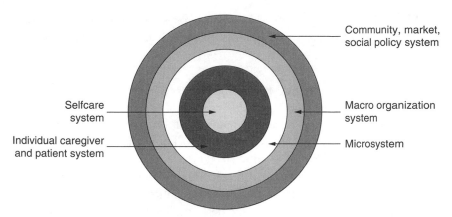

Community, market, social policy system

Selfcare system

Macro organization system

Individual caregiver and patient system

Microsystem

FIGURE 10–1. The systems of health care practice, intervention, measurement.

of caregivers responsible for a population of patients; beyond the microsystem lie the health care macrosystem and the larger community/economy within which the health care system resides.

Microsystem analysis recognizes that improvement in health care requires transformations at all levels of the health care system, but that ultimately the outcomes of larger health systems can be no better than the microsystems of which they are composed [1]. Moreover, the structure and functions of the caregiver portion of the microsystem should be determined by the characteristics of its patient population and the purposes for which they and the caregivers come together. For example, if a large proportion of the patient panel is young and many encounters are sports-related injuries, perhaps the caregiver team needs a physical therapist. If the majority of patients in the panel are monolingual in Spanish, the caregiver team needs many Spanish-speaking members. If diabetes, hypertension, and hyperlipidemia are common diagnoses in the patient panel, a priority might be a cardiovascular risk factor registry and chronic disease self-management training.

DIAGNOSING THE PRIMARY CARE MICROSYSTEM

The Dartmouth group has created many tools for diagnosing, or assessing, one's medical practice; they are available at: *www.clinicalmicrosystem.org*. A few of these tools are provided in Appendices B, C, D, E, G, and H.

Microsystem analysis divides the microsystem into four categories: patients, people, processes, and patterns. It is worth considering these in turn.

Who Are Your Patients?

The first step is learning about the patients. In order to prioritize problem solving in a microsystem, it is necessary to know the ten most frequent diagnoses of the patient population. If very few patients are children, it is probably not worth spending too much time on improving immunization practices and school physicals. If 20% of the patients have hypertension, it is extremely important to work on the best possible blood pressure management, including flow sheets, patient self-management support, and protocols allowing medical assistants—trained in hypertension management—to assist with their care. While these things seem obvious, many practices do not know how many patients they care for, the age, sex, and primary language distribution, or the ten more frequent diagnoses.

Another helpful exercise in *knowing your patients* is to list the 10 or 20 most frequent users of the practice. Every practice has some patients who make frequent appointments, drop in on a regular basis, and call the practice many times by phone. Some of these *frequent users* are very sick; others are not. These patients consume a disproportionate share of practice time, resources, and caregiver energy. It may be worthwhile to list them (any receptionist will immediately know who they are) and make a care plan for each of them. Perhaps a monthly hour-long visit with a nurse practitioner from the practice and home health nurse from a home health agency will do a great deal to help such a patient while reducing phone calls and drop-ins.

Who Are Your People?

A microsystem's people are the caregivers—the clinicians and staff. To help diagnose problems with caregivers, a central question is who does what? A useful microsystem tool is the activity survey. For each category (clinician, medical assistant, receptionist, and so forth) the survey asks what percent of time is spent doing what. For clinicians, activities include talking with patients, prescription refills, completing forms, different types of phone calls, evaluating test results, and looking for charts that are not available. If 20% of a clinician's time is spent leaving the exam room to find things and 10% is spent calling the hospital for lab and x-ray results, a major problem of wasted time has been uncovered. If the medical assistant spends 80% of her time putting patients in rooms and taking vital signs, she may be underutilized and could be trained to run the diabetes registry (see Chapter 4), help patients to develop behavior-change action plans, and follow up with patients about the plans (see Chapter 5). Periodically using a staff satisfaction survey (see Appendix E) can be an important step in building a cohesive clinical team.

What Are Your Processes?

Primary care microsystems engage in a number of regular processes, including registering patients, scheduling appointments, taking vital signs, rooming patients, diagnosing, treating, and counseling patients, receiving results from ancillary services and communicating these results to patients, refilling prescriptions, and billing and collections. Most processes are complex and involve more than one person. Flowcharts can be drawn to analyze the steps in each process, apportion the functions of each person in carrying out the steps of the process, and improving the hand offs between people. Flowcharts can help to uncover inefficiencies, delays, errors, and waste. Processes must be reconfigured when electronic innovations are introduced into a practice (see Chapters 7 and 8).

Perhaps the most helpful microsystem tool of all is the Assessment of Practice Processes (Appendix C), which elicits opinions on which processes work well, need repair, or are totally broken. At a staff meeting, each person in the practice can fill out the form; the practice leadership can add up the responses to determine which processes are priorities for improvement work. A helpful adjunctive tool provides a scatter diagram on which problems are more or less important, and which are easy or hard to fix. Ideally, a practice would start by improving a process that is (1) broken, (2) important, and (3) easy to fix.

Patients are a rich source of information for prioritizing which processes need the most attention. Satisfaction surveys can be collected by placing forms and a collection box in the waiting room. To be helpful, the questions asked need to be specific; for example, "How would you rate your ability to get through to the office by phone?" "Were you able to obtain your appointment in a timely fashion?" "Did you see the clinician or team member you wanted to see today?" "How would you rate your satisfaction regarding the time spent with the caregiver you saw today?" The surveys can be tailored to seek patient input on particular problems and proposed solutions (Appendix D).

What Are Your Patterns?

If 30% of the week's patient visits always occur on a Monday, that is a pattern. If 50% of the practice's patients with diabetes have Hb A1c levels greater than 7, that is a pattern. Patterns are analyses of practice data that can uncover problems [3, 4]. If only 2% of patients with diabetes have elevated Hb A1c levels, there is no significant problem. Patterns, then, are yet another method for diagnosing a microsystem.

Patterns can also suggest solutions to problems. If 30% of visits occur on Mondays, perhaps more staffing is needed on Mondays and more appointment slots need to be left open for the inevitable urgent phone calls and drop-ins (see Chapter 6). All the physicians taking vacations in August is a pattern, with an obvious (but not always easy to negotiate) solution. Income minus expenses over time are data that constitute a pattern; if income minus expenses is falling, this pattern uncovers a situation that goes to the top of the microsystem's problem list. To uncover patterns, microsystems need to take measurements.

Using the 4 P's to Diagnose a Microsystem

Taken together, the information gathered from the 4 P's (patients, people, processes, and patterns) provides a problem list—a list of diagnoses—for the microsystem. As with patients, diagnosis is not a one-time event. Over time, diagnostic workups continue at the same time as treatments are administered.

TREATING THE PRIMARY CARE MICROSYSTEM

Dr. Best decided to attend the Institute for Healthcare Improvement (IHI) conference on practice redesign. He was impressed by a workshop given by the Dartmouth group that developed microsystem analysis. He decided to try out some microsystem tools when he returned.

Dr. Best's practice includes four physicians, two nurse practitioners, four medical assistants, three receptionists, one medical records clerk, and two billing personnel. At an all-practice meeting, Dr. Best shared what he had learned at IHI, and an improvement team was chosen to lead a practice improvement effort. The team included Dr. Best, one nurse practitioner, one medical assistant, and one receptionist. Working with a small focus group of interested patients, the team made an initial diagnosis of the practice.

After prioritizing the problem list, the improvement team proposed four goals for the following 12 months. (1) Reduce the number of times clinicians are interrupted while seeing patients. (2) Improve the care of patients with diabetes so that the Hb A1c of 80% of the patients is below 7. (3) Guarantee that all patients receive an appointment within 1 week, and (4) Discuss behavior-change goals and action plans with at least 300 patients.

Once a practice sets performance goals, it is crucial to create systems of baseline and ongoing measurement [3, 4]. For the goal of reducing physician interruptions, clinicians can quickly record tic marks on the Unplanned Activity Tracking card (Appendix H), a simple microsystem tool; the numbers of interruptions per clinician can be tracked over time on a run chart publicly displayed in the practice waiting room. The diabetes goal is most easily measured by using a registry; in the absence of a registry, a manual system tracking Hb A1c levels can be created. For appointment delays, receptionists can record the time between a patient requesting and obtaining an appointment (see Chapter 6).

A practical construct for practice improvement is rapid cycle change, also known as the Plan-Do-Study-Act (PDSA) model [5]. This Model for Improvement was developed by a group of statisticians, inspired by Edward Deming, who helped revolutionize the Japanese (and as a consequence the U.S.) auto industry. The Model for Improvement has been used by IHI and many other organizations as a technique for making improvements in medical practices.

The Model for Improvement acknowledges that not all change creates improvement (some changes make things worse) and that concrete measurement is needed to demonstrate whether a change is an improvement. The model teaches people to ask themselves: What are we trying to accomplish (goals)? How will we know that a change is an improvement (by tracking data that measures achievement of the goals)? If a goal is to improve the glycemic control of patients with diabetes, a relevant measure is the percentage of people with diabetes who have Hb A1c levels of 7 or below.

Once the goals and measures are decided, the next task is to plan and implement a change that has the potential to create an improvement. This part of the model requires ingenuity—trying out something that might work, but abandoning plans that don't pan out in favor of something new. A central attribute of the Model for Improvement is impatience—try out the change today or tomorrow. Traditionally, changes involve 90% planning and 10% (or 0%) implementation. Under the PDSA method of the Model for Improvement, a plan is quickly made (Plan), it is immediately implemented as a test with perhaps one physician and three patients (Do), the test is analyzed to see what worked and what did not (Study), and the plan is changed to make it work better (Act = new Plan). Then a second, presumably better, PDSA is done. Once the change works well with the one physician and three patients, it can be spread to more physicians and patients.

An example: Dr. Best's fourth goal—discussing behavior-change goals and action plans with at least 300 patients. A PDSA cycle might start by training one physician to engage three patients in discussing behavior-change goals and action plans (Plan). The next day, the physician is trained and discusses goal setting and action plans with three patients (Do). After getting feedback from the physician the improvement team concludes that the goal-setting discussions took an average of 7 minutes each, too long to incorporate into the 15-minute office visit (Study). A new plan is developed to train one medical assistant to do goal-setting discussions with three patients. The physician would briefly explain the process to the patient, and if the patient agrees, the medical assistant would have the goal-setting discussion (Act = Plan-2). This second PDSA cycle was tried the following day (Do-2). By the third patient, the medical assistant felt comfortable discussing action plans, but patient flow was disrupted because the medical assistant spent 20 minutes with each patient (Study-2). A schedule was worked out that the medical assistant would conduct goal-setting discussions on Wednesdays and Thursdays, the days with the fewest patients, so that another medical assistant could handle the patient flow for two clinicians (Act-2 = Plan-3) This time, the plan worked. After 2 weeks the plan was spread to two more physicians and one more medical assistant. New kinks were worked out using the PDSA method. The medical assistants were responsible to fill in a large thermometer chart showing how many patients had been engaged in behavior-change goal setting. The improvement team also decided that the medical assistants would follow up on patients' action plans by phone every 2 weeks. This additional work required more PDSA cycles because the time required for follow-up necessitated the reduction of other medical assistant functions that were found to be nonessential. Every 3 months, a few patients who had made behavior-change goals and action plans were invited to evaluate the process in meetings with the improvement team.

The PDSA method contrasts with traditional improvement methods, which involve detailed planning—often by managers with little frontline involvement—and the promulgation of a policy change, which is launched for all clinicians and all patients without the PDSA emphasis on pilot testing. The traditional method can waste much time developing the complexities of a plan, seeking buy-in from a number of people, and possibly scrapping the entire change if it fails to work. In contrast, the rapid cycle concept wastes no time testing and evaluating a change with one clinician and a few patients, and tweaking the change with repeated PDSA cycles until implementation can take place on a broader scale.

CONCLUSION

Problems in primary care practices, whether sites in integrated delivery systems or small family physician offices, can be addressed by forming an improvement team; assessing (diagnosing) the microsystem; prioritizing the problems uncovered by patients, staff, and clinicians; setting measurable goals and creating data systems to track goal achievement; initiating PDSA cycles to test changes; and following the data to make sure that the changes truly represent improvement. At the same time, the improvement team needs to periodically monitor staff responses to staff satisfaction surveys, understanding that quality, productivity, financial stability, and patient satisfaction are closely tied to staff cohesion. In the case of Dr. Best, the improvement process has transformed him from an attitude of coping to one of mastering his work. Starting with small, solvable problems creates a climate of success that catalyzes further improvement.

REFERENCES

1. Nelson EC, Batalden PB, Huber TP, et al: Microsystems in health care: Part 1. Learning from high-performing front-line clinical units. J Comm J Qual Improv. 2002;28:472–493.
2. Buckingham M, Coffman C: *First, Break All the Rules*: What the World's Greatest Managers Do Differently. New York, Simon and Schuster, 1999.
3. Nelson EC, Batalden PB, Homa K, et al: Microsystems in health care: creating a rich information environment. Jt Comm J Qual Saf. 2003;29:5–15.
4. Nelson EC, Splaine ME, Batalden PB, et al: Building measurement and data collection into medical practice. Ann Intern Med. 1998;128:460–466.
5. Langley GJ, Nolan KM, Nolan TW, et al: *The Improvement Guide.* San Francisco, CA, Jossey-Bass, 1996.

CHAPTER ELEVEN

Payment for Primary Care

Dr. Edward Lo, a family physician, was upset. It had been a hard month. The home visits to the two patients who had died were necessary and professionally satisfying, but had taken a lot of time, as had the multiple calls coordinating care with the home care nurses and the family. Four patients had required emergency surgery necessitating urgent calls to surgeons, faxing medical records, coordinating with hospitalists; as a result, on 4 separate days the office was justifiably in chaos with everything running 2 hours behind. Yet the revenue took another dip and the staff had just received a raise at the same time that health insurance premiums for the staff jumped 18%.

At the medical staff meeting that night Dr. Lo sat next to the chief of radiology. "We're so glad to have you here referring all those ultra-sounds and MRI (magnetic resonance imaging) scans to us. Each of our three radiologists topped $300,000 last year and we're grateful."

Dr. Lo liked the specialists on the hospital staff. They were of high quality and he could not practice medicine without them. But he felt that the income disparity between family physicians and specialists was unfair

The Medical Group Management Association (MGMA) conducts yearly surveys of physician compensation [1]. Table 11-1 shows the median 2004 compensation for a number of specialties, along with the 5-year and 10-year change in compensation. For primary care as a whole, median pretax income increased by 21.4% from 1995–2004, compared with a 37.5% increase for non–primary care specialties. While 50% of family physicians made below $156,000 in 2004, half of all radiologists earned above $407,000 in that year. The growing income gap between primary care physicians and specialists is confirmed by other data sources [2–4].

TABLE 11–1
Changes in physician compensation by specialty

Median Compensation, 1995–2004. MGMA data	1995	2000	2004	10-year change 1995–2004	5-year change 2000–2004
All primary care:	**$133,329**	**$147,232**	**$161,816**	21.4%	9.9%
Family practice (without OB)	$129,148	$145,121	$156,011	20.8%	7.5%
Internal medicine	$139,320	$149,104	$168,551	21.0%	13.0%
Pediatric/ adolescent medicine	$129,085	$141,676	$161,188	24.9%	13.8%
All specialists:	**$215,978**	**$256,494**	**$297,000**	37.5%	15.8%
Anesthesiology	$240,666	$280,353	$325,999	35.5%	16.3%
Cardiology: invasive	$337,000	$365,894	$427,815	26.9%	16.9%
Cardiology: noninvasive	$239,406	$300,073	$351,637	46.9%	17.2%
Dermatology	$176,948	$213,876	$308,855	74.5%	44.4%
Emergency medicine	$176,439	$198,423	$221,679	25.6%	11.7%
Gastroen-terology	$209,913	$281,308	$368,733	75.7%	31.1%
Hematology/ oncology	$188,569	$258,403	$350,290	85.8%	35.6%
Neurology	$164,295	$175,143	$211,094	28.5%	20.5%
Obstetrics/ gynecology	$215,000	$223,207	$247,348	15.0%	10.8%
Ophthalmology	$209,736	$236,353	$280,353	33.7%	18.6%
Orthopedic surgery	$301,918	$335,646	$396,650	31.4%	18.2%
Otorhino-laryngology	$220,000	$235,415	$296,623	34.8%	26.0%

TABLE 11–1 Changes in physician compensation by specialty (*Continued*)					
Median Compensation, 1995–2004. MGMA data	**1995**	**2000**	**2004**	**10-year change 1995– 2004**	**5-year change 2000– 2004**
Psychiatry	$132,477	$156,486	$182,799	38.0%	16.8%
Pulmonary medicine	$170,529	$195,557	$230,688	35.3%	18.0%
Radiology: diagnostic	$247,505	$298,824	$406,852	64.4%	36.2%
Surgery: general	$216,562	$245,541	$282,504	30.4%	15.1%
Urology	$213,448	$301,772	$335,731	57.3%	11.3%

Source: Ref. 1

THE PRIMARY CARE-SPECIALTY INCOME GAP

The Resource-Based Relative Value Scale (RBRVS) system was designed by William Hsiao and associates at the Harvard School of Public Health [5, 6]. RBRVS was adopted by Medicare in 1992, and forms the basis of many private insurance companies' physician payment methods.

Dr. Lo sees an established patient with diabetes, hypertension, and stable angina for 30 minutes. According to the Medicare fee schedule, the 2005 fee for this extended office visit (Current Procedural Terminology— CPT—code 99214) is $89.64. The fee is calculated by multiplying the Relative Value Unit (RVU) for a 99214 CPT code by the conversion factor for 2005, and adjusting the fee according to the geographic locality of the physician. In 2005, the RVU for a 99214 visit was 2.18; the conversion factor for all CPT codes was 37.9. Thus $2.18 \times 37.9 = \$82.62$. This number is adjusted upward because Dr. Lo's practice is in Chicago where practice expenses are above average; in Nebraska the same service would garner a fee of $76.74. CPT codes for office and hospital visits, both for primary care physicians and specialists, are called evaluation and management (E/M) codes.

Dr. Samuel Scopes performs a colonoscopy in a Chicago hospital endoscopy suite. The procedure takes 30 minutes. A colonoscopy, CPT code 45378, has an RVU of 5.46. Multiplying by the same 37.9 conversion factor and adjusting for the geographic location, the Medicare fee is $226.63.

Why is the gastroenterologist paid so much more than the family physician for the same 30 minutes of work?

While interviewing a number of physicians during the 1980s, Dr. Hsiao concluded that practice expense and work performed were the major factors that should determine payment. Practice expense for different specialties could be computed from physicians' tax returns. Several factors were incorporated into the calculation of work performed: time, mental effort and judgment, technical skill and physical effort, and psychological stress. Dr. Hsiao conducted telephone interviews of a random sample of physicians in a number of specialties, asking the physicians to estimate the amount of work required to furnish different services or to perform different procedures. Based on the results of these interviews, he assigned work values to different services and procedures. These values became the work portion of the RVUs in the RBRVS system [5].

A 30-minute office visit pays less than a 30-minute colonoscopy because the physicians surveyed by Dr. Hsiao estimated that the mental effort and judgment, technical skill and physical effort, and psychological stress was greater for procedural work than for office visit work. Hsiao's methodology helps to explain the gap between the incomes of procedural specialists and primary care physicians. But there is a conundrum. The RVU values of many procedure codes have gone down in relation to the value of E/M codes. In 2000, a colonoscopy fee was 342% of a 99214 office visit while in 2005, the colonoscopy was worth 247% of a 99214 visit. While many procedural and imaging RVU values have increased over time, coronary artery bypass surgery RVU values have decreased as have the values for cholecystectomy, colectomy, breast surgery, and a number of other diagnostic and surgical procedures.

Why, then, has the gap between procedural specialists and primary care physicians continued to widen?

THE KEY ROLE OF VOLUME

Dr. Scopes was not pleased. His colonoscopy fee was a bit lower in 2004 compared with 2001. He believed that fees should go up, not down. He decided to give family practice grand rounds at three hospitals on the role of colonoscopy in colon cancer screening. Two months later, he was getting many new referrals. He was now doing 15 colonoscopies each week rather than the 10 he had averaged before. Things were going well.

In 1988, in a commentary on the publication of the RBRVS system, the administrator of the federal Medicare program predicted that specialists whose fees were reduced by RBRVS were likely to respond by increasing the volume of procedures they performed [7]. This prediction has come true as the volume of procedures performed by specialists has grown substantially [8, 9].

A 2005 report by the Urban Institute detailed the average annual change in the volume of services per Medicare beneficiary by specialty from 1998 to 2002 [10]. While family practice volume grew by 2.6% and internal medicine by 3.6% per year, cardiology increased by 5.9% annually, orthopedic surgery by 4.2%, and dermatology by 5.9%. Thoracic surgery volume did not increase, and general surgery volume grew by only 1.5% [11].

The primary care–specialty gap has increased at different rates for different specialties. The ratio of family practice to general surgery income was .6 in 1995 and .55 in 2004, a relatively small change related to reductions in both the fee and the volume of common surgeries performed by general surgeons. In contrast, the family practice-radiology ratio dropped from .52 in 1995 to .38 in 2004. Radiologists enjoyed huge growth in volumes of services provided.

Some volume data are available for the entire adult population, not restricted to Medicare beneficiaries. The number of office visits to family practice and internal medicine physicians per adult population did not increase from 1993 to 2000 [11, 12]. In contrast, the number of angioplasties per adult population increased by 45% during those years; hip replacements increased by 25%, knee replacements by 86%, and laparoscopic cholecystectomies by 56%. Coronary artery bypass surgeries, however, decreased by 10% [13].

To uncover the significance of volume in determining income, another clue may reside in data showing increases in productivity by specialty. Productivity—a marker for volume of services provided—can be measured in a number of ways: numbers of visits or procedures per physician per year, numbers of RVUs per physician per year, or gross charges—the amount billed for services provided—per physician per year. Using gross charges for all payers (Medicare, Medicaid, private insurers, and patient self-pay), data from the MGMA allows a comparison between increases in income growth and volume growth [1].

The MGMA data shows that six specialties demonstrated the greatest percentage increase (over 40%) in income from 1994 to 2004: noninvasive cardiology, dermatology, gastroenterology, hematology/oncology, diagnostic radiology, and urology. Five of these six specialties are among the list of seven specialties with the highest (over 80%) increase in productivity during those 10 years. In other words, there is a close association between increasing volume and increasing income, suggesting that changes in volume may be more significant than changes in fee levels in determining income growth.

By becoming more efficient in performing procedures (fewer minutes per procedure), specialists can increase their volume without increasing the time they spend in patient care. In contrast, primary care physicians cannot reduce the time per office visit without reducing quality and patient satisfaction (see Chapter 1); primary care physicians cannot produce more RVUs without working more hours.

Trapped in this way, many primary care practices are adding office-based diagnostic tests or minor procedures to boost their income [14]. A number of these add-ons are cosmetic or of questionable medical value, cannot be considered as true primary care, and reduce physician time available for primary care services. Other primary care practices are supplementing insurance payments with retainers from patients through the institution of boutique or concierge practices. While these solutions are understandable in the current environment, neither is consistent with the mission of high-quality primary care accessible to the entire population.

FEE-FOR-SERVICE PAYMENT AND THE NEW PRACTICE MODEL

RVU values and volumes account for differential incomes between primary care physicians and specialists. This income gap contributes to the dearth of U.S. medical school graduates choosing primary care careers (see Chapter 1). Lower primary care incomes, particularly when combined with growing practice expenses, leave primary care practices without the funds needed to invest in practice innovation and computerization.

The quantity of primary care payment is one barrier to the development of the New Practice Model described in Chapter 2. Another perhaps greater barrier is the manner in which most primary care practices are reimbursed. Fee-for-service payment of clinicians (physicians, nurse practitioners, and physician assistants) performing face-to-face visits is the dominant way in which Medicare, Medicaid, and commercial insurers pay primary care practices. Planned chronic care visits by nurses or pharmacists (see Chapter 4) and self-management support activities conducted by nonclinicians (see Chapter 5) are often unpaid and thus not financially viable.

WHAT COULD BE DONE TO CHANGE THE SITUATION?

In 1999, the *New England Journal of Medicine* published an article which criticized the RBRVS methodology estimating physician work according to time, mental effort and judgment, technical skill and physical effort, and psychological stress. The article claimed that the duration of the face-to-face encounter with the patient or family (whether for office visits or procedures) is strongly predictive of the amount of work performed, calling into question the other determinants of the work portion of the RVU in the RBRVS system [15]. If RVU values were assigned purely by time spent, primary care work would increase substantially in value compared with specialty procedures.

Such a reform would not solve the primary care–specialty gap created by increasing procedural and imaging volumes. Confronting the volume problem would require analysis of the appropriateness of services performed by different physicians in different metropolitan areas, with payment withheld for inappropriate services.

To create incentives for the New Practice Model, substantial reform of the mode of payment is necessary. Team-based care, with nonclinicians taking responsibility for a number of primary care functions (see Chapters 2 and 9), requires payment of nonclinicians for the time they spend with patients. Such payment could be in the form of adequate capitation, fees for nonclinician visits, a care management payment for patients with chronic conditions, or pay-for-performance bonuses that are far larger than those currently paid under most current performance-based schemes. In addition, telephone and electronic encounters can substitute for face-to-face visits only if they are financially rewarded.

Primary care physicians need to press their professional associations to take bold positions on primary care payment—both the amount of payment and the manner in which primary care practices are paid. This includes mobilizing the public, whose members want their own personal primary care physician, and educating budget-minded political and business leaders who do not yet understand that only a primary care–based system can control health care costs.

REFERENCES

1. Data furnished by Medical Group Management Association, Englewood, CO, December 2005.
2. Crane M: Survey Report earnings: time to call a code? Medical Econ. 2001 (September 17);18:74.
3. Lowes R: The earnings freeze. Medical Econ. 2005 (September 16);82:58.
4. Center for Studying Health System Change: *Physician Survey*. Washington, DC, 1996–2001. *(http://CTSonline.s-3.com/psurvey.asp)*
5. Hsiao WC, Braun P, Yntema D, et al: Estimating physicians' work for a resource-based relative-value scale. N Engl J Med. 1988;319:835–841.
6. Hsiao WC, Dunn DL, Verrilli DK: Assessing the implementation of physician-payment reform. N Engl J Med. 1993;328:928–933.
7. Roper WL. Perspectives on physician payment reform. N Engl J Med. 1988;319:865–867.
8. Medicare payment to physicians. Statement of Glenn Hackbarth, November 17, 2005. Medicare Payment Advisory Commission (MedPAC). (*www.medpac.gov*)
9. Healthcare Spending and the Medicare Program. A Data Book. Medicare Payment Advisory Commission (MedPAC), June 2005. (*www.medpac.gov*)
10. Maxwell S, Zuckerman S, Aliaga P: *Effects of the Implementation of Resource-Based Practice Expense Relative Value Units Under the Medicare Fee Schedule*, 1998–2002. Washington, DC, The Urban Institute, March 2005.
11. Cherry DK, Woodwell DA: *National Ambulatory Medical Care Survey: 2000 Summary*. DHHS Publication 02-0379. Hyattsville, MD, National Center for Health Statistics, May 2002.
12. Woodwell DA, Schappert SM: *National Ambulatory Medical Care Survey: 1993 Summary*. DHHS Publication 6:0029. Hyattsville, MD, National Center for Health Statistics, December 1995.
13. *Health, United States, 2004*. Hyattsville, MD, National Center for Health Statistics, 2004.
14. Weiss GG: Adding ancillaries: boosting the bottom line. Medical Econ. 2005 (November 4);82:98.
15. Lasker RD, Marquis MS. The intensity of physicians' work in patient visits. N Engl J Med. 1999;341:337–341.

CHAPTER TWELVE

Conclusion

In January 2009, Dr. Ernesto Futuro was named Secretary of Health and Human Services. For the preceding 23 years, Dr. Futuro had been a family physician in El Paso, Texas, working in a two-physician office with a general internist. Dr. Futuro was deeply concerned with the future of primary care. He believed in the New Practice Model of primary care and had mixed success implementing new model components into his own practice. He did not feel it was possible to spread the new models across the country one practice at a time. He believed that innovation within each microsystem was necessary, but that a national health policy was needed at the macrosystem level to assist primary care practices in adopting the new models.

Dr. Futuro spent his first 6 months educating members of Congress, the newly elected President, state governors, and large employers about the value of primary care, particularly emphasizing its ability to reduce health care costs. He carefully studied and adopted policy recommendations from the American Academy of Family Physicians, American College of Physicians, and Society of General Internal Medicine [1–5]. Dr. Futuro felt that primary care could be rescued with a three-pronged approach: creating a new way of paying for primary care, assisting primary care practices to create functioning teams that could improve care and make life easier for clinicians, and elevating the stature of primary care in medical schools.

In mid-2009, Dr. Futuro, with the President's support, persuaded several members of Congress to introduce a package of bills related to primary care. One bill mandated Medicare to make a fundamental change in how primary care was to be reimbursed. Primary care practices would receive payment through multiple mechanisms: a fixed sum for practice expenses, a capitation payment for each Medicare patient enrolled, a fee *for specific preventive services, bonuses for high quality and prompt access, and a care coordination payment for patients with chronic illness. The care coordination payment would support primary care practices in hiring nonphysician caregivers to provide self-management support and planned care for patients with chronic conditions. Medicare would also contribute funds to primary care computerization. These payment increases would be financed by reductions in overpriced procedural and imaging services, by the reduced number of hospital admissions and emergency department visits resulting from stronger primary care, and by a national program of post-hospital heart failure care estimated to reduce Medicare hospital expenditures by billions of dollars.*

Dr. Futuro had worked with promotoras (community health workers) in Texas, and felt that they could help with patient self-management support, interpreter services, and sustained follow-up of chronic conditions. He arranged for a national promotora bill that would provide funds for community colleges to train promotoras and would partially subsidize primary care practices to hire promotoras. He also promoted legislation to extend medical school loan forgiveness to all students entering primary care careers.

Dr. Futuro encouraged the formation of a "Rescue Primary Care Coalition," led by the American Academy of Family Physicians, American College of Physicians, Society of General Internal Medicine, American Academy of Pediatrics, American Academy and American College of Nurse Practitioners, American Academy of Physician Assistants, American Association of Medical Colleges, the National Association of Community Health Centers, and the National Association of Public Hospitals and Health Systems. The coalition also included some specialty societies that understood how a vibrant primary care sector would relieve specialists of responsibilities they did not want.

Dr. Futuro spoke at the Annual Conference of the Nation's Governors about the importance of state legislation to legalize the provision of routine preventive and chronic care by nonclinician caregivers using protocols or standing orders from physicians.

By 2011, all the primary care bills had become law, and a number of states had passed legislation extending the scope of services that could be provided by nonclinician caregivers with physician-written protocols and close physician supervision.

The results were dramatic. Although the new models of primary care practice had been limited to a small number of innovators, the new payment mechanisms galvanized most practices to adopt new model components.

Other insurance plans followed suit in implementing Medicare's new primary care payment policies. The excitement within medical schools and nonphysician clinician training programs was palpable. The number of students choosing primary care careers doubled. In response to the demand of primary care practices for promotoras and other nonclinician caregivers, slots in training programs for these careers multiplied.

Dr. Futuro left the government in 2012. He was determined to spend a few years back at his El Paso medical office. He wanted to see how it felt to practice in the new primary care friendly environment.

REFERENCES

1. Future of Family Medicine Project Leadership Committee: The future of family medicine. Ann Fam Med. 2004;2(Suppl 1):S3–S32.
2. American Academy of Family Physicians: *The New Model of Primary Care: Knowledge Bought Dearly.* 2004. *(http://www.aafp.org/PreBuilt/caremanagementpolicy.pdf)*
3. American College of Physicians: *The Advanced Medical Home: A Patient-Centered, Physician-Guided Model of Health Care.* 2006. *(http://www.acponline.org/ hpp/adv_med.pdf)*
4. American College of Physicians: *The Impending Collapse of Primary Care Medicine and Its Implications for the State of the Nation's Health Care.* 2006. *(http://www.acponline.org/hpp/statehc06_1.pdf)*
5. Society of General Internal Medicine: *The Future of General Internal Medicine.* 2003. *(www.sgim.org/futureofGIMreport.cfm)*

Some Organizations and Resources Demonstrating Innovative Primary Care Practices

Group Health Cooperative of Puget Sound has made great progress in chronic care management (the Chronic Care Model was developed at Group Health's Center for Health Studies), organization of primary care teams, and electronic access by patients to their medical chart and their care team via the Internet. For a demonstration of Group Health's electronic patient portal, go to *www.ghc.org* and click on MyGroupHealth Demo.

Kaiser Permanente has done some of the best improvement work on chronic disease management. Information on some of its programs is available at the Web site of Kaiser Permanente's Care Management Institute (*www.kpcmi.org*).

HealthPartners Medical Group in Minnesota is one of the most innovative delivery systems in the nation. The organization has pioneered improvements in chronic care, implemented advanced access, and published numerous articles exploring the facilitators and barriers to primary care

194   Appendix A

improvement through its HealthPartners Research Foundation (*www.health-partners.com*).

Harvard Vanguard Medical Associates was an early adopter of the electronic medical record, and like Group Health has an electronic patient portal allowing patients to get lab results, ask questions, schedule appointments, and renew prescriptions (*www.harvardvanguard.org*).

Palo Alto Medical Foundation in northern California has an electronic medical record and an electronic patient portal with health education modules, a summary of each medical visit, and capability for prescription refills, obtaining lab results, making appointments, and e-mailing information to the care team. In addition, the organization has considerable experience offering group visits (*www.pamf.org*).

CareSouth Carolina in Hartsville, South Carolina, is a community health center with multiple sites in poor, rural areas. The health center has made marked improvements in chronic care outcomes for its patients, using planned visits with care managers who work with patients to improve their self-management skills (*www.caresouth-carolina.com/innovations.asp*).

Clinica Campesina, a community health center serving largely uninsured Latino patients in Denver, Colorado, has introduced multiple innovations including advanced access scheduling, improvements in diabetes and asthma outcomes, group visits, and well-developed primary care teams (*www.clinicacampesina.org*).

Greenfield Health System in Portland, Oregon, is a laboratory for many primary care innovations. The practice is a leader in substituting e-visits in place of many face-to-face visits (*www.greenfieldhealth.com*).

The Alaska Native Medical Center, through a commitment to patient-centered care, has successfully developed primary care teams, high-quality chronic care management, same-day access, and telemedicine/telepharmacy to serve remote villages. A description is available at *www.ihi.org* (enter Alaska Native Medical in the search box on the upper right of the home page).

Charles Burger, MD, has created a state-of-the art private practice in Bangor, Maine, including a smoothly functioning health care team in which every person in the practice has clear tasks and responsibilities and team members communicate electronically with one another.

The State of Wisconsin has a number of innovative primary care practices including ThedaCare Physicians, Bellin Medical Group, Gundersen Lutheran Health System, and Marshfield Clinic. Measures of timely access to appointments, chronic illness care, patient satisfaction, and more are available for several of these practices on the Web site of the Wisconsin Collaborative for Healthcare Quality (*www.wchq.org*).

Case studies on innovative practices are available in a book by S Houck (Houck S. *What Works: Effective Tools and Case Studies to Improve Clinical Office Practice*. Boulder, CO, HealthPress Publishing, 2004).

The Institute for Healthcare Improvement Web site has many case reports of innovative primary care practices (*www.ihi.org*). Click on Topics, then Office Practices, and under each subtopic look for improvement stories at the bottom of the page.

The American Academy of Family Physicians is piloting a Practice Enhancement Program to teach small- and medium-sized practices how to implement practice improvements. More information is available at *www.aafp.org/pep.xml*

The American College of Physicians is starting a Center for Practice Innovation to disseminate practice redesign strategies for small- and medium-sized practices. More information is available at *www.acponline.org/cfpi/*

The American College of Physicians also published a 2006 document on the *Advanced Medical Home. (http://www.acponline.org/hpp/statehc06. htm)*.

Assessing your Practice

Introduction

Clinicians work hard in today's health care environment. Finding the time and tools to critically reflect and analyze practice is hard. This workbook is a *map* that can be customized to local context and needs in order to support practice evaluation and improvement. Identification of *broken* processes, wastes and delays, and deeper knowledge of patients and people can improve patient care, outcomes, and staff work life.

Aim

Provide an organized, locally adaptable method to assist practices in collecting information and data to identify opportunities that can lead to significant improvements that improve patient care, outcomes, and staff work life.

A. Know Your Patients (Practice Profile)   See Items: ❶ ❷ ❸

Understand the needs of your patient

- ❏ Estimate the number of patients in your practice
- ❏ List the age distribution of patient population
- ❏ List percentage of females
- ❏ List your practice's top 10 conditions
- ❏ List your top 10 *high utilizers*
- ❏ Measure daily demand
- ❏ List the number of patients seen in a day
- ❏ List the number of patients seen in the last week
- ❏ List the number of new patients in the last month
- ❏ List other clinical microsystems you regularly interact with

- ❏ List health outcome measures
- ❏ List the number of dis-enrolling patients in the last month
- ❏ List encounters per provider per year. Attach a separate list of the providers with actual number of encounters per year. If part-time provider, annualize the number.
- ❏ Measure patient satisfaction
- ❏ Note the number of out-of-practice visits which occur each year: condition sensitive hospital rate and emergency room visit rate
- ❏ Utilize *www.howsyourhealth.org*

B. Know Your People (Practice Profile)   See Items: ❹ ❺

Assess your personnel

- ❏ Identify members of staff (*Add additional page if necessary*)
- ❏ Identify FTE by member (*Clarify clinical time vs. other responsibilities*)
- ❏ Define roles
- ❏ List hours of operation
- ❏ Measure daily capacity
- ❏ Measure backlog (*Third available appointment*)

- ❏ List current appointment types and duration
- ❏ List services currently offered, e.g., group visits, e-mail, patient web site, etc.
- ❏ Measure staff satisfaction
- ❏ Note if every member of the practice meets regularly
- ❏ Note your operating margin (revenue minus expense)
- ❏ Evaluate individual skills and needs

C. Know Your Processes (Activity Surveys, Occurrence Tracking, Telephone Logs, Unplanned Activities, Walk-through worksheet)
See Items: ❻ ❼ ❽ ❾ ❿ ⓫ ⓬ ⓭ ⓮ ⓱

- ❏ Measure office visit cycle time (patient cycle tool - sample 1 day of patients which includes all providers)
- ❏ Complete activity survey sheets (per staff member)
- ❏ Complete telephone tracking log (1 week)
- ❏ Complete demand (specialty) tracking log (1 week)
- ❏ Complete nurse triage tracking sheet (1 week)

- ❏ Track visit and non-visit activities occurrences (1 week)
- ❏ Track unplanned activities (sample 1 day for provider)
- ❏ Complete a *walk-through* of your practice from the patient perspective
- ❏ Complete the practice core and supporting process assessment.

D. Know Your Patterns (Practice Profile, Patient Satisfaction Survey, Patient Cycle Tool)   ❶ ❷ ❹ ⓫ ⓬ ⓯ ⓰ ⓲ ⓳ ⓴

- ❏ Third available appointment by provider (backlog)
- ❏ Office visit cycle time (patient cycle tool)
- ❏ Daily demand
- ❏ Daily capacity
- ❏ Patient satisfaction
- ❏ Staff satisfaction
- ❏ Assessment tool for core/key processes

- ❏ Operating margin
- ❏ Note if every member of the practice meets regularly
- ❏ List things you are most proud of
- ❏ List things you have successfully changed
- ❏ Identify how safety and reliability issues are discussed
- ❏ Strategize improvement based on assessments
- ❏ Outcome measures

NOTE: We have developed this workbook with tools to give ideas to those interested in improving health care. "Dartmouth- Hitchcock Medical Center and the developers of this workbook are pleased to grant use of the these materials without charge, providing that recognition is given for their development, that any alterations to the documents for local suitability and acceptance are shared in advance, and that the uses are limited to their own use and not for resale."

Diagnosing Problems in your Practice

- Adapt the list of processes to your practice. Distribute the evaluation form to all practice staff. Tally the results to give the Lead Team data on where to begin improvement.

- **Steps for Improvement:** Explore improvements for each process based on the outcomes of this assessment tool. Each of the processes below should be flowcharted in its current state. Once you have flowcharted the current state of your processes and determined your change ideas, use the Plan-Do-Study-Act Cycle Worksheet to run tests of change.

Primary Care Practice: Know Your Processes (Core and Supporting Processes)							
Processes	Works well	Small problem	Real problem	Totally broken	Cannot rate	We're working on it	Source of patient complaint
Answering phones							
Appointment system							
Scheduling procedures							
Order diagnostic testing							
Reporting diagnostic test results							
Prescription renewal							
Making referrals							
Preauthorization for services							
Billing/coding							
Phone advice							
Assignment of patients to your practice							
Orientation of patients to your practice							
New patient work-ups							

Primary Care Practice: Know Your Processes (Core and Supporting Processes) (*Continued*)							
Processes	Works well	Small problem	Real problem	Totally broken	Cannot rate	We're working on it	Source of patient complaint
Minor procedures							
Education for patients/ families							
Prevention assessment/ activities							
Chronic disease management							

Primary Care Patient Survey

Today's Office Visit

Please rate the following questions about the visit you just made to this office.

	Excellent	Very Good	Good	Fair	Poor
1. The amount of time you waited to get an appointment	☐	☐	☐	☐	☐
2. Convenience of the location of the office	☐	☐	☐	☐	☐
3. Getting through to the office by phone	☐	☐	☐	☐	☐
4. Length of time waiting at the office	☐	☐	☐	☐	☐
5. Time spent with the person you saw	☐	☐	☐	☐	☐
6. Explanation of what was done for you	☐	☐	☐	☐	☐
7. The technical skills (thoroughness, carefulness, competence) of the person you saw	☐	☐	☐	☐	☐
8. The personal manner (courtesy, respect, sensitivity, friendliness) of the person you saw	☐	☐	☐	☐	☐
9. The clinician's sensitivity to your special needs or concerns	☐	☐	☐	☐	☐
10. Your satisfaction with getting the help that you needed	☐	☐	☐	☐	☐
11. Your feeling about the overall quality of the visit	☐	☐	☐	☐	☐

General Questions

Please answer the general questions about your satisfaction with this practice.

12. If you could go anywhere to get health care, would you choose this practice or would you prefer to go someplace else?
☐ This practice ☐ Someplace else ☐ Not sure

13. I am delighted with everything about this practice because my expectations for service and quality of care are exceeded.
☐ Agree ☐ Disagree ☐ Not sure

14. In the last 12 months, how many times have you gone to the emergency room for your care?
☐ None ☐ Once ☐ Twice ☐ Three or more

15. In the last 12 months, was it always easy to get a referral to a specialist when you felt like you needed one?
☐ Yes ☐ No ☐ Does not apply

16. In the last 12 months, how often did you have to see someone else when you wanted to see your personal doctor or nurse?
☐ Never ☐ Sometimes ☐ Frequently

17. Are you able to get to your appointments when you choose?
☐ Never ☐ Sometimes ☐ Always

18. Is there anything our practice can do to improve the care and services for you?
☐ I'm satisfied ☐ Improve some things ☐ Improve many things
Specify improvement:

19. Did you have any good or bad surprises while receiving your care?
☐ Good ☐ Bad ☐ No surprises
Please describe:

About You

20. In general, how would you rate your overall health?
☐ Excellent ☐ Very good ☐ Good ☐ Fair ☐ Poor

21. What is your age?
☐ Under 25 years ☐ 25–44 years ☐ 45–64 years ☐ 65 years or older

22. What is your gender?
☐ Female ☐ Male

Primary Care Staff Satisfaction Survey

1. I am treated with respect every day by everyone who works in this practice.

☐ Strongly agree   ☐ Agree   ☐ Disagree   ☐ Strongly disagree

2. I am given everything I need—tools, equipment, and encouragement—to do my work.

☐ Strongly agree   ☐ Agree   ☐ Disagree   ☐ Strongly disagree

3. When I do good work, someone in this practice notices that I did it.

☐ Strongly agree   ☐ Agree   ☐ Disagree   ☐ Strongly disagree

4. How stressful would you say it is to work in this practice?

☐ Very stressful   ☐ Somewhat stressful   ☐ A little stressful   ☐ Not stressful

5. How easy is it to ask anyone a question about the way we care for patients?

☐ Very easy   ☐ Easy   ☐ Difficult   ☐ Very difficult

6. How would you rate other people's morale and their attitudes about working here?

☐ Excellent   ☐ Very good   ☐ Good   ☐ Fair   ☐ Poor

7. This practice is a better place to work than it was 12 months ago.

☐ Strongly agree   ☐ Agree   ☐ Disagree   ☐ Strongly disagree

8. I would recommend this practice as a great place to work.

☐ Strongly agree   ☐ Agree   ☐ Disagree   ☐ Strongly disagree

9. What would make this practice better for patients?

_____

10. What would make this practice better for those who work here?

_____

Resources on Cultural Competence and Health Literacy

King T, Wheeler M, Bindman A, et al (eds.): *Medical Management of Vulnerable and Underserved Patients: Principles, Practice and Populations.* New York, McGraw-Hill, 2006.

Smedley BD, Stith AY, Nelson AR, (eds.): *Unequal Treatment: Confronting Racial and Ethnic Disparities in Health Care.* Washington, DC, National Academies Press, 2003.

Fadiman A: *The Spirit Catches You and You Fall Down: A Hmong Child, Her American Doctors, and the Collision of Two Cultures.* New York, Farrar, Straus, and Giroux, 1997.

National Center for Cultural Competence at Georgetown University. (*http://gucchd. georgetown.edu/nccc/*)

American Medical Student Association has a good Web site on cultural competence in medicine. (*www.amsa.org/programs/gpit/cultural.cfm*)

Department of Health and Human Services Office of Minority Health has a Center for Linguistic and Cultural Competence in Health Care. (*www.omhrc.gov*)

University of Washington Harborview Medical Center in Seattle has created an excellent Web site. (*www.ethnomed.org*)

The journal Family Practice Management has a cultural competence self-test: Sutton M: Cultural competence. Fam Pract Manag. October 2000. (*www.aafp.org/fpm/20001000/58cult.html*)

The American Association of Medical Colleges has produced a booklet on cultural competence education for medical students. (*www.aamc.org/meded/ tacct/culturalcomped.pdf*)

The Kaiser Family Foundation has put together a compendium of cultural competence initiatives in health care. January 2003. (*www.kff.org/uninsured/ 6067-index.cfm*)

A review of evidence on the effects of limited health literacy. (*www.ahrq.gov/clinic/ epcsums/litsum.htm*)

The California Health Literacy Initiative Web site contains a wealth of information and resources on health literacy training and materials for patients. (*www.cahealthliteracy.org*)

Office Visit Cycle Time

DEFINITION

The office visit cycle time is the amount of time in minutes that a patient spends in an office visit. The cycle begins at the time of arrival and ends when the patient leaves the office. (Note: The cycle time does not include time spent in laboratories or radiology during primary care visits. Specialty clinics may opt to include testing and procedure times in total cycle time since these activities are an integral part of the planned specialty care visit.)

Both primary care and specialty clinics may wish to distinguish between the time the patient spends with the physician or other members of the care team (*value-added* time) and the time spent waiting (*non–value-added* time). The goal is not to reduce total cycle time but to maximize the time the patient spends with the physician or other members of the care team.

GOAL

Decrease the office visit cycle time to 30 minutes or 1.5 times the actual time spent with clinician. For example, if the average patient spends 20 minutes with a clinician during the office visit, then the goal for the office visit cycle time would be 30 minutes (1.5×20 minutes = 30 minutes).

DATA COLLECTION PLAN

Sample a minimum of 15 patients per week on a preselected day and time. Use the same day and time of day each week. Selecting a time during the day that is often the busiest in the office is a good method to ensure that the data capture the true capability of the system. If the patient arrives early, time starts at scheduled time of appointment. The patient takes the cycle time form with him/her throughout the visit and records the time that each part of the visit begins (e.g., time the patient checks into the appointment desk, the time in the waiting room, the time in the exam room, the time spent with the clinician, the time spent in post-visit activities, the time while checking out, and the time the patient leaves the office).

These materials were adapted from Institute for Healthcare Improvement and the Center for the Evaluative Clinical Sciences at Dartmouth. *(www.ihi.org/IHI/Topics/OfficePractices) and (www.clinicalmicrosystem.org)*

Primary Care Practice Patient Cycle Time					
		Day:		Date:	
Scheduled appointment time			Provider you are seeing today		
Time					
		1.			
		2.			
		3.			
		4.			
		5.			
		6.			
		7.			
		8.			
		9.			
Comments:					

Interruptions in the Day's Work

- Patterns can offer hints and clues to our work that inform us of possible improvement ideas. The Unplanned Activity Tracking Card is a tool you can ask staff to carry to track patterns of interruptions, waits, and delays in the process of providing smooth and uninterrupted patient care. Start with any group in the staff. Give each staff member a card to carry during a shift, to mark each time an interruption occurs when direct patient care is delayed or interrupted. The tracking cards should then be tallied to review possible redesign opportunities.

Primary Care Practice: Unplanned Activity Tracking Card							
Unplanned activity tracking				**Unplanned activity tracking**			
Name:				Name:			
Date:		Time:		Date:		Time:	
Place a tally mark for each occurrence of an unplanned activity			**Total**	**Place a tally mark for each occurrence of an unplanned activity**			**Total**
Interruptions				Interruptions			
• Phone				• Phone	ḤḤ ḤḤ ḤḤ		⑮
• Secretary				• Secretary			
• RN				• RN	ḤḤ ḤḤ		⑩
• Provider				• Provider			
Hospital admissions				Hospital admissions	ḤḤ ḤḤ ll		⑫
Patient phone calls				Patient phone calls			
Pages				Pages	ḤḤ ḤḤ ḤḤ ḤḤ		20
Missing equipment				Missing equipment			
Missing supplies				Missing supplies	ḤḤ		5
Missing chart: same day patient				Missing chart: same day patient			
Missing chart: patient				Missing chart: patient	ḤḤ ḤḤ		⑩
Missing test results				Missing test results			
Other				Other			

Group Visit Starter Kit*

WHAT IS A GROUP VISIT?

The term is applied to visits designed for groups of patients, rather than individual patient-provider appointments. This starter kit describes the Cooperative Health Care Clinic (CHCC) model developed by the Kaiser Colorado staff. We will refer to it simply as a group visit. Group visits were pioneered with elderly patients who were high utilizers of primary care.

In this model, the health care team facilitates an interactive process of care delivery in a periodic group visit program. The team empowers the patient, who is supported by information and encouraged to make informed health care decisions. The group visit can be conceptualized as an extended doctor's office visit where not only physical and medical needs are met but educational, social, and psychological concerns can be dealt with effectively.

Invitations are extended by the health care team to specific patients on the basis of chronic disease history and utilization patterns. The patients typically remain in the same group together. Members may be added to groups if the group size decreases. Variations of this group visit format have been used for disease or condition specific populations, such as diabetes, hypertension, orthopedic procedures, heart failure, cancer, asthma, depression, hormone replacement, and chronic pain.

---

*www.improvingchroniccare.org

Some groups begin with monthly meetings and later adjust to quarterly. Some clinics find it helpful to provide a group meeting periodically for new patients as an orientation to the clinic, or to initiate a new clinical guideline. Another group visit model, Drop-In Group Medical Appointments (DIGMA), follows a different methodology and is not discussed here.

PLANNING AND IMPLEMENTING GROUP VISITS

Two months before the first group visit

It is important to begin planning at least 2 months before the first visit is scheduled to occur. Make sure that you have support from the leadership at your site. Discuss with the leadership what outcomes you want from your group visits. Some suggestions include patient and provider satisfaction, achievements on clinical standards of care, and utilization. Determine a measurement plan.

At a team meeting, determine the population you would like to invite for group visits. Remember that 30–50% of patients are amenable to participation in group appointments, so determine if the population you wish to include has at least 50 patients or the group that results from your invitation may be too small to make the visit efficient for your team. Chronic illness registries and reports of patients with frequent visits can be used for this purpose. At this first team meeting, review the letters of invitation, standard agenda for the first meeting, and the roles of the team members. A task list and timeline are provided in the following section. Give top priority to scheduling the primary care provider, the nurse, and a medical assistant (MA) to assist with vitals during the break in the group visit. Don't forget to schedule the room.

One month before the first group visit

When a list of potential patients is obtained, the team should quickly review the list for patients who wouldn't be appropriate in a group. The typical exclusions are patients who are terminally ill, have memory problems, severe hearing problems, have difficulty with English (unless you are offering a second language session), or are out of the area for significant portions of the year. Create your mailing list and letters now. Plan to have letters reach patients about 1 month before the first session. The letter is viewed most positively if it is personally signed by the primary care provider, and followed up 1 or 2 weeks after the mailing with a personal phone call from the nurse who will be attending the group visits.

It is a good idea to have a second team meeting during this time. The materials for the patients to have at the first session should be reviewed. They should be provided with a folder or three-ring binder to bring with them on each visit. Review any assessments or documentation tools you wish to use. Discuss how the calling is going (or went) and who is expected to attend. Review the agenda and roles of the team. Some clinics like to provide coffee or a snack for the break in the visit. Arrange this as needed, as well as the materials for the folders, binders, a flip chart, BP cuffs, and stethoscopes. It is a good idea to use nametags, especially for the first few visits.

One week before the first group visit

About 1 week before the first session, enlist someone to call the attendees and remind them of their appointment. These calls should describe the purpose of the visit, what is likely to occur at the visit, and encourage the patient to attend. The caller should reinforce that this is an actual medical appointment, not a class or workshop, and people are expected to call and cancel if they cannot attend. Discuss the issues of co-pay and parking as necessary. Many teams request the charts of those who will be attending and review them for preventive care needs or other concerns.

Supplies for a group visit
Charts
BP cuffs and stethoscopes
Specialty Tools (e.g., monofilaments for diabetes foot exam)
Forms (sign-in sheets, order forms, and the like)
Pens
Nametags
Flip charts and markers

Day of the first group visit

On the day of the first session, prepare the room well in advance, as some patients will arrive early. Tables should be set up in the shape of a horse-shoe with the open end pointing toward the speaker. Start on time to create the expectation that the visit has a beginning and an ending. At least one team member should be in the room to greet patients. Help patients to write the name they wish to be called by in large letters on their name tag.

Don't hog the airtime!
If the facilitator has been talking about himself/herself for more than 1 minute, it's time to stop!

The primary care provider should open the meeting on a welcome note. All staff and team members should be introduced and the patients should be given a format to follow for introductions. It is important to include sharing in the introduction, as this will help to form the supportive relationships between the group members. For older patients, reminiscence can be very helpful. The primary care provider should model the introduction. The provider should introduce himself/herself again using the exact format he/she wants the participants to use. For example, "My name is (use the name you wish to be addressed by). My favorite childhood toy was my bicycle. We used to ride all around our neighborhood in Des Moines, Iowa on our bikes." This modeling will help other participants to be brief. If participants begin to tell extended stories, the provider might need to interrupt gently by saying something like "Thank you, ——. We need to make sure we have time to hear from everyone." The introductions should take about 15 minutes.

After the introductions, the provider gives an overview of the group visit (30 minutes). Allow lots of time for interaction and questions. Review the group norms, which cover the expectation of confidentiality for the group.

We all like food
Consider offering simple refreshments. In some groups, the members will take on the responsibility and offer to bring items to share.

Before the break, the provider and nurse should explain what will happen. The nurse will start at one end of the horseshoe and take vitals and the physician will start at the other end and cover any individual issues. Some groups have found it helpful to have a medical assistant take vitals in addition to the nurse. Vitals are recorded for the patients in their notebooks, and for the medical record. All team members should assess patients for those who may need an individual visit at the end of the group session.

After the break (15 minutes), the group should reconvene for an open question and answer period. The provider may need to prompt this session and encourage participation at first. Often asking what people have heard or seen on the news or in the newspaper will get the questions rolling. The provider should involve the team as much as possible and refer questions to the nurse to demonstrate to the patients that the team works together.

After the question and answer period, the group discusses what topic they would like to discuss in the next group visit (typically 1 month in the future). Writing down a list of all the ideas on a flip chart can be a very helpful technique. Providers find that patients typically bring up topics that the provider team also feels are important and rarely suggest frivolous topics. If they do, other participants usually discourage the idea. Some provider teams may want to get a quick reaction from the participants about what they liked about the meeting. The participants are thanked for attending the session.

Let the group answer questions
When questions arise, health care professionals tend to want to give the answers. Instead, learn to leverage the power of the group. "Has anyone else experienced this problem? What worked for you?" This increases the participants' confidence in their own problem-solving ability.

Individual appointments then follow at 10-minute intervals. The nurse and provider may both have individual appointments. After 30 minutes of appointments, the provider is rewarded for the group visit by having 30 minutes of discretionary time.

After the first group visit, the team may want to have a short debriefing meeting. Discuss what went well and what didn't go so well. As you discuss things you might want to do differently, remember that the basic format of the group has been tested in clinical trials, and deviations from the outline may not have the same positive results.

Providers have found that few materials should be prepared in advance of the group visit. Quickly reviewing the patient information materials your clinic usually uses is generally all that is required. What the patients want to hear is the basic information they need to know and how others have dealt with the situation. Providers should strive for each session to be interactive.

WHO DOES WHAT

Each team should review the tasks and roles and determine how best to use their team. The result might look something like this:

LPN/MA

1. Pull charts 3–5 days before the group visit
2. Remind primary care provider about the upcoming group visit
3. As agreed upon by team, perform chart review
4. Give results of chart review to provider

Day of Group visit

1. Check room setup
2. Take charts and supplies to room
3. Perform vitals, exams, and immunizations as needed
4. Data entry into registry, if appropriate

Appointing Personnel

1. Reminder phone calls to patients
2. Check on room reservation
3. Make sure name tags are ready

Day of Group Visit

1. Prepare charts and labels

2. Print out registries for patients, if appropriate

3. Complete billing information as needed

MD

1. Participate in planning of the visit with the team, following suggestions of participants

2. Review charts, identify problems for review with individual patients

Day of Group Visit

1. Conduct discussion and group visit

2. During break, review individual needs and make 1:1 individual appointments for after the visit

3. Document all visits

RN

1. Coordinate the planning of the visit with the team

2. Coordinate materials and information for the visit

Day of Group Visit

1. Circulate in room during break, performing vital signs, and identifying patients who need individual attention

2. After visit, follow up with patients via telephone as needed

Others: pharmacist, behavioral health, nutrition, physical therapy

It is helpful to provide access to other caregivers during the group visits. Discourage guest presenters from lecturing to the patients or providing them with excessive prepared materials. A good model for these presentations is for the physician, nurse, or presenter to have the group list all the questions they have before the presenter speaks. If these are listed on a flip chart, they can be checked off as they are discussed.

LETTER INVITING PATIENTS TO GROUP VISITS

Date

Dear

I want to invite you to participate in a new way of delivering medical care. This program is designed specifically for (*describe group:* patients with _____ and patients over 65). By choosing to participate you will be asked to:

- Become a member of a small group of patients with ————. This group will meet every month with me to address medical and other issues of concern to you.

- Help us develop the program for your particular group.

- Help evaluate the success of the program in meeting your needs.

Most of the time when you come in to the clinic, you are ill or have a specific problem that we need to talk about. Discussions about managing or improving your health are often hard to fit into these short visits. The purpose of this group is improved health. In the group, we will discuss ways you can maintain or improve your health and make sure you are up to date with care recommended for you.

The first group visit will be held _____ (day and date) from _____ (A.M. or P.M.). These group visits will be held at _____. We encourage you to bring a family member with you. Since this visit includes a medical evaluation, a co-pay will be collected if you usually pay for medical care.

If you are interested, please RSVP by _____ (date) to _____ (name) at _____ (phone number). If you are not interested, you will continue to receive usual health care.

Sincerely,

_____

Primary care clinician

Task list and timeline				
Date	**Action**	**Responsibility**	**Done**	**Comments**

Two months before first session

    Meet with leadership

    Determine goals and
      measurement

    Team meeting (1 hour or less)
      Determine type of group visit
      (e.g. elderly)
      Discuss plans and team
      member roles
      Review agenda and letters

    Schedule room (2-hour block)

    Schedule provider (2-hour block)

    Schedule RN (2-hour block)

    Schedule MA for vitals
    during break

    Obtain list of potential participants

    Review list for inappropriate
    invitees

One month before first session

    Send out invitation letters to
    40–50 people

    Call all patients who received
    letter (2 weeks after mailing)

    Team meeting (45 minutes
    or less)

      Review agenda and roles,
      attendees, patient notebooks

    Arrange refreshments, if desired

    Create records for patients
    (folder/notebook 25 per group)

One week before

    Create roster of attendees and
    sign-in sheet

    Review charts for potential
    immediate needs

    Call attendees to remind them
    of their appointment

Task list and timeline				
Date	Action	Responsibility	Done	Comments
Day of visit				
	Set up room (horseshoe)			
	Materials in room (patient folders, coffee, BP cuffs, stethoscopes, flip chart, nametags, tissues)			
	Be in room early to greet patients			
	Hold visit			
	Debrief after visit:			
	What went well? What didn't go as well?			
Monthly				
	Plan next group visit			

GROUP VISIT NORMS

We will...

- Encourage everyone to participate.
- State our opinions openly and honestly.
- Ask questions if we don't understand.
- Treat one another with respect and kindness.
- Listen carefully to others.
- Respect information shared in confidence.
- Try to attend every meeting.
- Be prompt, so meetings can start and end on time.

AGENDA FOR FIRST SESSION

15 minutes	**Introductions/Welcome:** Physician opens the session. Team members present are introduced. Introductions follow around the room, with sharing included. Example for older patients: Give your name as you would like to be called, and share your favorite childhood game or favorite childhood holiday memory, and so forth.
30 minutes	**Group Visits:** What are they? Why are we doing it? What should you expect? Questions from the group. Group visit norms. Review folder/notebook.
15 minutes	**Break:** Physician starts on one side, nurse on the other.
	Take blood pressures; ask about specific concerns for the day (look for patients who need 1:1 visits). Refill meds.
15 minutes	**Questions and Answers:** Ask for any questions the group has about their health, the visit, and so on.
15 minutes	**Planning:** Topic for next month. Announce time and date.
30 minutes	**1:1 visits with provider and nurse as needed**
30 minutes	**Provider discretionary time**

AGENDA TEMPLATE

15 minutes	**Introductions/Welcome**
	Physician opens the session.
	All team members present are introduced.
	Introductions follow around the room, with sharing included.
30 minutes	**Topic of the Day**
	Physician and nurse provide information, interacting with the participants, whenever possible. Some suggestions to make the session interactive include asking:
	"Has anyone here ever had this problem?"
	"How has anyone dealt with this situation before?"
	"What have you heard about _____?"
	Intersperse the presentation with questions from the group
15 minutes	**Break**
	Physician starts on one side, nurse on the other.
	Take blood pressures, ask about specific concerns for the day (look for patients who need 1:1 visits), refill meds.
15 minutes	**Questions and Answers**
	Ask group for questions about their health, the visit, recent topics in the news.
15 minutes	**Planning and Closing**
	Determine topic for next month. Thank everyone for coming.
30 minutes	**1:1 visits with provider and nurse**
30 minutes	**Provider discretionary time**

Source: Improving Chronic Illness Care is a national program supported by The Robert Wood Johnson Foundation with direction and technical assistance provided by Group Health Cooperative's MacColl Institute for Healthcare Innovation.

Resources Available from Improving Chronic Illness Care

Health care organizations require practical assessment tools to guide quality improvement efforts and evaluate changes in chronic illness care. In response to this need, the ICIC staff developed the Assessment of Chronic Illness Care (ACIC) survey. The content of the ACIC was derived from specific evidence-based interventions for the six components of the Chronic Care Model. The ACIC can be downloaded from *www.improvingchroniccare.org*.

Once an organization undertakes an improvement effort, the clinicians involved will need tools to assist in changing care for their patients.

The following tools can be downloaded from *www.improvingchroniccare.org*.

- Condition-Specific Resource Guides and Collaborative Training Manuals
- Group Visit Starter Kit
- Delivery System Design: Comparison of Group Visit Models
- Comparison of Four Diabetes System Innovations
- Red-Yellow-Green (a.k.a *Stoplight*) Tools for Patients
- Condition-Specific Resources for Children's Health Care

227

- Planned Asthma Care (PAC) Self-Management Manual
- Continuing Care Clinic Handbook
- Self-Management Support: Patient-Planning Worksheet
- Depression Management Tool
- Bureau of Primary Health Care Recommended System Requirements for Vendors of Electronic Patient Care Systems
- Information about Registry Comparison
- Registry Product Evaluation Tool
- Card File Registry
- Diabetes Eye Exam Report
- Foreign Language Diabetes Education Materials

RESOURCES FOR PEOPLE WITH CHRONIC ILLNESS

MEDLINEplus at the National Library of Medicine (NLM) at the National Institutes of Health (NIH).   MEDLINEplus brings together, by health topic, authoritative information from NLM, the NIH, and other government, nonprofit, and health-related organizations. It also provides a database of full text drug information and an illustrated medical encyclopedia.

National Center for Chronic Disease Prevention and Health Promotion at the Centers for Disease Control.   Information about chronic diseases and conditions, lists of publications from the National Institutes of Health, and links to other sources of health information, health and education agencies, major voluntary associations, the private sector, and other federal agencies.

InfoNet.   InfoNet, from Johns Hopkins Medical Institutions, offers an extensive list of advocacy and self-help organizations, and Web sites on chronic diseases and aging that are searchable by condition.

Partnership for Solutions.   A chronic conditions–oriented Web site, developed by Johns Hopkins University and The Robert Wood Johnson Foundation, to communicate research findings to policymakers, business leaders, health professionals, advocates, and others. The site contains chart books, research syntheses, and other aids that can be useful in describing the issues faced by the chronically ill.

American Cancer Society.   This site provides information on prevention (including diet, smoking avoidance, exercise, alcohol intake, and hormones), risk factors, mammograms, breast self-exams, and treatment options.

American Diabetes Association.   This site has an online postgraduate course for health care professionals. There is little patient education material. You can search by state for local diabetes foundations, research, and resources, some of which do have a fair amount of patient education material.

American Heart Association.   There is an index of nearly 300 subjects from the American Heart Association (AHA). Information on nutrition, exercise, and support groups is included. There is a listing of books and cookbooks available for purchase from the AHA.

American Lung Association.   This contains patient education materials on lung health and disease. This information is intermingled with links to information about the association itself, so it may be difficult to sort out the patient education materials.

Arthritis Foundation.   This is a very comprehensive site. Different types of treatment and causes of arthritis are included. There are links to 200 local chapters of the foundation, as well as information on ordering video and audio tapes and other materials. There are also free brochures available.

Internet Resources for Health Education and Health Promotion. This site contains a selected bibliography of Internet resources on health education and promotion. It was compiled by the George Washington University Medical Center.

National Cancer Institute. From the home page, click on Cancer Information for education materials on cancer for patients, health professionals, and basic researchers.

National Diabetes Education Program. The National Diabetes Education Program has compiled a resource to help health care professionals deliver the ongoing patient-centered care required to effectively manage diabetes. This Web site is designed for primary care providers, diabetes educators, specialists, and organizations. It provides steps, models, guidelines, resources, and tools for the process of making and evaluating effective systems change.

National Digestive Diseases Information Clearinghouse. This site includes information for patients and health care practitioners on diabetes, digestive diseases, endocrine diseases, kidney diseases, nutrition and obesity, and urologic diseases.

National Heart, Lung, and Blood Institute. This site contains information on diseases affecting the lungs, blood, and sleep disorders.

National Institute of Arthritis and Musculoskeletal and Skin Diseases. This site contains information on fibromyalgia, Lyme disease, lupus, psoriasis, Raynaud's phenomenon, vitiligo, and other skin, arthritic, and musculoskeletal diseases.

National Guideline Clearinghouse. Consumer information on specific health conditions, surgery, prescriptions, health plans, and other health care issues. Start your search by typing keywords into the search box on this page, or click on the *NGC Resources* tab on the left, top side of the home page.

Nutrition World Wide Web from University of Arizona. Catalog, nutrition-related publications, and links.

Source: Improving Chronic Illness Care is a national program supported by The Robert Wood Johnson Foundation with direction and technical assistance provided by Group Health Cooperative's MacColl Institute for Healthcare Innovation.

Patient Assessment of Chronic Care

Patient Name: _____

Caregiver Name: _____   Date: _____

Staying healthy can be difficult when you have a chronic condition. We would like to learn about the type of help you get with your condition from your health care team. This might include your regular doctor, his or her nurse, or physician's assistant who treats your illness. Your answers will be kept confidential.

Over the past 6 months, when I received care for my chronic conditions, I was:

		Never	Rarely	Sometimes	Frequently	Nearly always
1.	Asked for my ideas when we made a treatment plan.	0	1	2	3	4
2.	Given choices about treatment to think about.	0	1	2	3	4
3.	Asked to talk about any problems with my medicines or their effects.	0	1	2	3	4
4.	Given a written list of things I should do to improve my health.	0	1	2	3	4
5.	Satisfied that my care was well organized.	0	1	2	3	4
6.	Shown how what I did to take care of myself influenced my condition.	0	1	2	3	4
7.	Asked to talk about my goals in caring for my condition.	0	1	2	3	4
8.	Helped to set specific goals to improve my eating or exercise.	0	1	2	3	4
9.	Given a copy of my treatment plan.	0	1	2	3	4
10.	Encouraged to go to a specific group or class to help me cope with my chronic condition.	0	1	2	3	4

Over the past 6 months, when I received care for my chronic conditions, I was:					
	Never	Rarely	Sometimes	Frequently	Nearly always
11. Asked questions, either directly or on a survey, about my health habits.	0	1	2	3	4
12. Sure that my doctor or nurse thought about my values, beliefs, and traditions when they recommended treatments to me.	0	1	2	3	4
13. Helped to make a treatment plan that I could carry out in my daily life.	0	1	2	3	4
14. Helped to plan ahead so I could take care of my condition even in hard times.	0	1	2	3	4
15. Asked how my chronic condition affects my life.	0	1	2	3	4
16. Contacted after a visit to see how things were going.	0	1	2	3	4
17. Encouraged to attend programs in the community that could help me.	0	1	2	3	4
18. Referred to a dietitian, health educator, or counselor.	0	1	2	3	4
19. Told how my visits with other types of doctors, like an eye doctor or surgeon, helped my treatment.	0	1	2	3	4
20. Asked how my visits with other doctors were going.	0	1	2	3	4

Source: Improving Chronic Illness Care is a national program supported by The Robert Wood Johnson Foundation with direction and technical assistance provided by Group Health Cooperative's MacColl Institute for Healthcare Innovation.

Self-management Support Tools

Sample dialogue to assess importance and confidence

Caregiver: I just got back your last Hb A1c; it rose to 8.5

Patient: It's supposed to be 7 or lower

Caregiver: That's right. What would you like to do?

Patient: I'm already on a diet, and I'm so busy, I have no time for exercise. I don't know what to do.

Caregiver: Could we talk a bit about the exercise?

Patient: Umm, yeah, OK

Caregiver: How important is it to you to increase your exercise? Let's do this on a scale of 0–10. A 0 means it isn't important, and 10 means it's just about as important as it can get.

0 1 2 3 4 5 6 7 8 9 10
Not important   Important

Patient: It's an 8. I know I really need to do it.

Caregiver: Now, using the same 0–10 scale, how confident are you that you can get more exercise? A 0 means you aren't sure at all, 10 means you're 100% sure.

0	1	2	3	4	5	6	7	8	9	10

Not sure   Very sure

Patient: It's a 4. Like I said, I have no time.

Caregiver: Why did you say 4 and not 1?

Patient: I can exercise on the weekends, so it's not something that's completely impossible.

Caregiver: What would it take to raise the confidence level of a 4 to an 8?

Patient: Maybe if I could exercise with a friend, I'd enjoy it more, be more motivated. I have a friend at work who has diabetes too.

Caregiver: Do you want to set a short-term goal about your exercise? We could agree on an action plan.

Lessons from the dialogue. The caregiver allows the patient to approve the agenda, "Could we talk a bit about the exercise?"

If level of importance is high, 7 or above, the caregiver moves on to confidence level. If level of importance is low, it may help to provide more information about the risks of not changing the behavior. In that case, the caregiver might propose an action plan, for example, "Would you like to read this pamphlet about diabetes and talk about it the next time I see you?"

If the level of confidence is medium-low (e.g., 4), the caregiver asks why it is 4 and not 1. That puts the patient in a position to speak positively about why there is *some* level of confidence.

Asking what it would take to change the 4 to an 8 makes the patient think creatively about how to make a behavior change. In this case, it leads to an action plan. The action plan might be to talk to the friend at work tomorrow and ask about exercising together—an achievable action plan that could lead to a further action plan (e.g., to walk with the friend for 20 minutes at lunch on Mondays, Wednesdays, and Fridays).

If there is a sufficient level of importance and confidence to make a behavior change, the caregiver suggests discussing an action plan. Some practitioners of motivational interviewing feel that action plans are only appropriate if readiness to change (importance and confidence) is high; others believe that action plans can be discussed at any level of importance and confidence, but that the action plans must be tailored to the importance and confidence levels.

If patients or caregivers have difficulty working with 0–10 scales, other ways of demonstrating importance and confidence can be used, such as thumbs-up or thumbs-down pictographic scales .

Agenda-setting dialogue

Caregiver: Your hemoglobin A1c has gone up from 7.5 to 8.5.

Patient: That's not good, it's supposed to be under 7.

Caregiver: Would you like to spend a few minutes discussing what we might do?

Patient: OK.

Caregiver: Let me ask you this, do you have any idea about how you might bring your Hb A1c back down?

Patient: Well, probably the way I eat, do exercise, and take my pills have a lot to do with it.

Caregiver: That's right. We have a tool called a bubble chart that has some choices for improving your Hb A1c. Is there anything on this chart you might like to focus on?

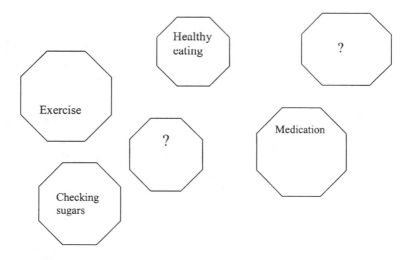

Patient: I think I'd like to talk about exercise.

Ask-tell-ask dialogue

Caregiver: I just checked your blood sugar and I have to tell you something very important. You have diabetes.

Patient: Diabetes? Oh my god!

Caregiver: Do you know what diabetes is? [ASK]

Patient: I know someone who had it, her blood sugar went way up and she went into a coma and died.

Caregiver: A coma is actually very rare in your kind of diabetes.

Patient: Another person I know had to get his toe cut off. He also had major trouble with his eyes.

Caregiver: Those things can happen in diabetes, but they can also be prevented. Tell me this; what would you like to know about diabetes [ASK]?

Patient: I need to know how to keep my feet attached to my body.

Caregiver: Why don't we spend the next half hour talking about how to prevent the serious complications of diabetes. Is that OK?

Patient: Let's get started.

[A 30-minute informational session: TELL]

Caregiver: Next visit I'm going to ask you what you remember from our discussion. Is there anything else you would like to do in the next visit [ASK]?

Closing-the-loop and shared decision-making dialogue

Caregiver: You have been trying very hard to improve your diet and exercise, but your Hb A1c has only come down from 10 to 8.5. I would recommend that we try to bring it down below 7. What do you think?

Patient: If it will keep my feet attached to my body, let's go for 7.

Caregiver: Your choices are to make your diet even stricter, do even more exercise, or start taking a medication called Metformin. [Shared decision making requires offering choices]

Patient: I think we need to go for the medicine.

Caregiver: OK. [Explains about Metformin: what it does, possible side effects] I would suggest we start with one pill twice a day. If you start having problems with your stomach or bowels, cut down to once a day for a week and then go back to twice a day.

Patient: OK.

Caregiver: Let's just make sure I was clear in what I said. Can you tell me how you will be taking your Metformin?

Patient: Twice a day no matter what.

Caregiver: What if you have problems with your stomach or bowels?

Patient: Oh, yes. Twice a day but go down to once a day for a week if I feel problems.

Caregiver: Great! The medical assistant will be calling you in a week to see how you are doing.

Goal-setting dialogue

Caregiver: Your last lab test shows your Hb A1c has gone up to 9.2. What do you think about that?

Patient: I don't know. I'm taking my pills. I thought if I took them I didn't have to worry about eating candy and sweets every day; the pills are supposed to protect me.

Caregiver: What is it you like about eating candy?

Patient: I love chocolate; it's kind of comforting, I have all these things that stress me out, but I know that chocolate is one thing in my day I will definitely enjoy.

Caregiver: That makes sense. Is there anything you don't like about eating chocolate?

Patient: Well, it messes up that sugar. But I don't want to give it up, like I said- it makes me happy.

Caregiver: Is there anything else you enjoy doing that reduces your stress but doesn't get your Hb A1c so high?

Patient: Maybe walking around the block a couple of times.

Caregiver: Do you want to give that a try?

Patient: Sure, but I'm not promising to give up chocolate.

Caregiver: I understand. Let's do a reality check? How sure are you that you can walk around the block a couple of times when you feel stressed? Let's use a 0–10 scale: 0 means you aren't sure you can succeed and 10 means you are very sure you can succeed.

Patient: I can do it; I'm 100% sure.

Caregiver: Let's try to make this as specific as possible. Rather than walking every time you feel stressed, how about walking two times around the block every day after lunch?

Patient: Well, if I feel stressed, that might be OK.

Caregiver: Why don't we call it your action plan—you will walk around the block two times when you feel the stress coming on. When do you want to start?

Patient: We'll see.

Caregiver: Do you want to start this week?

Patient: That might work

Caregiver: OK. Why don't we agree that you will walk around the block two times when you feel stress? Could I call you next week to see how it's going?

Patient: OK.

Lessons: When the patient mentions an unhealthy behavior (chocolate), the caregiver doesn't challenge it, but uses a motivational interviewing technique: what do you like and what don't you like about the unhealthy behavior. This encourages the patient, not the caregiver, to talk about change (what he/she *doesn't* like). This may uncover a topic for an action plan—in this case, relieving stress.

The caregiver does not judge the patient's behavior. When the patient says, "I'm not promising to give up chocolate," the caregiver doesn't make a judgment, but says, "I understand," and moves on.

The action plan should be simple and specific. The 0–10 scale estimates the patient's confidence that he/she can succeed at the action plan. The purpose of the action plan is to *increase self-efficacy* (self-confidence that the patient can change something). The goal is success. It doesn't matter how small the behavior change is; the important thing is that the patient succeeds, thereby increasing self-efficacy. To maximize the chance of success, the patient should have high confidence, at least 7 out of 10, that he/she can succeed. If, for example, a sedentary patient proposes an action plan to walk 5 miles a day, with a low-level confidence (2 out of 10) that he/she can succeed, the caregiver should suggest a more achievable action plan.

At the end of the dialogue, the caregiver tries to make the action plan more specific ("When do you want to start?"), but the patient resists ("we'll see" and "that might work"). Rather than challenging the patient, the caregiver *rolls with the resistance* and goes with what the patient is willing to do. Sometimes the patient will not want to make an action plan at all.

Problem solving (when making a follow-up phone call)

1. Identify the problem (the most difficult and important step).

2. List ideas to solve the problem.

3. Pick one, try it for two weeks.

4. Assess the results.

5. If it doesn't work, try another idea.

6. Utilize other resources (family, friends, professionals).

7. If nothing seems to work, accept that the problem may not be solvable now.

Problem-solving methods are provided in a book by Lorig and Holman. (Lorig, Holman, et al: *Living a Healthy Life with Chronic Conditions.* Boulder, CO, Bull Publishing, 2006.)

Self-management Support Assessment

1. Does your practice have a systematic process to screen or assess patients for the following risk factors?

	Yes, electronic only	Yes, paper or paper and electronic	No	Don't know
a. Smoking/tobacco use	❏	❏	❏	❏
b. Obesity/weight management	❏	❏	❏	❏
c. Alcohol/substance abuse	❏	❏	❏	❏
d. Depression	❏	❏	❏	❏
e. Dementia	❏	❏	❏	❏

2. Does your practice provide written, audio, video, or web-based patient instructions or educational materials that are appropriate for the language needs of at least 90% of patients?

	Yes	No	Don't know
a. Written materials	❏	❏	❏
b. Audio	❏	❏	❏
c. Video	❏	❏	❏
d. Web-based	❏	❏	❏

3. Does your practice provide for or refer patients to formal support programs to assist in self-management for conditions or age-specific risk factors? Formal programs include classes or programs. Do not count guidance during a regular office visit and provision of brochures.

	Provides	Refers	Neither	Don't know
a. Smoking cessation	❏	❏	❏	❏
b. Substance abuse	❏	❏	❏	❏
c. Weight loss or management	❏	❏	❏	❏
d. Nutrition	❏	❏	❏	❏
e. Physical activity	❏	❏	❏	❏
f. Asthma	❏	❏	❏	❏
g. Diabetes	❏	❏	❏	❏
h. Cardiovascular disease	❏	❏	❏	❏
i. Depression	❏	❏	❏	❏
j. Other conditions (specify_____)	❏	❏	❏	❏

4. Does your practice routinely use the following activities to encourage patient self-management?

	Yes	No	Don't know
a. Provide a plan that includes patient preferences, goals, and action plans	❏	❏	❏
b. Provide a convenient method for recording and reporting self-monitoring results	❏	❏	❏
c. Provide written materials that explain to patients the guidelines for recommended medical care for their illness (e.g., guidelines for retinopathy for patients with diabetes)	❏	❏	❏
d. Give specific instructions on when and how to seek emergency care	❏	❏	❏
e. Assist patients in identifying and overcoming barriers to adherence	❏	❏	❏

5. For what conditions does your practice have systems to encourage patient self-management?

	Yes	No	Don't know
a. Diabetes	❏	❏	❏
b. Cardiovascular disease	❏	❏	❏
c. Depression	❏	❏	❏
d. Asthma	❏	❏	❏
e. Other condition	❏	❏	❏

Review of Evidence on the Chronic Care Model

This informal review summarizes studies on three of the four Chronic Care Model elements that are internal to the primary care practice. Evidence for self-management support is reviewed in Chapter 5.

DECISION SUPPORT

The two major components of decision support are clinical practice guidelines and physician education. Simply making clinical practice guidelines available to physicians does not change medical practice [1]. Some forms of physician education can improve physician performance and (less frequently) clinical outcomes. Continuing medical education conferences and printed educational materials for physicians are not effective, while academic detailing (outreach visits by physician educators) is usually successful. Interactive educational workshops for physicians improve medical practice while didactic presentations have little effect. Combining several educational interventions produces a greater proportion of positive changes in health outcomes than using a single intervention [2–5].

A review of 12 studies of physician education in managing hypertension—including continuing medical education classes, computerized decision support systems, printed educational materials, and academic detailing—concluded that physician education alone was ineffective in improving blood pressure levels [6].

A systematic review of 70 studies concluded that availability of decision support as part of clinician workflow and at the time and location of decision making, and computer-based decision support, were associated with improved clinical practice [7].

DELIVERY SYSTEM REDESIGN: PLANNED VISITS

Diabetes

In Kaiser Permanente's trial of planned group diabetes visits led by a nurse educator, group visit participants had significantly reduced Hb A1c levels and lower hospital use compared with controls [8]. Peters and Davidson demonstrated that patients attending a nurse-led diabetes planned visit clinic had improved Hb A1c levels that were lower than those of usual care patients [9]. Aubert came to similar conclusions [10].

Planned telephone encounters by nurses between primary care office visits were associated with improved Hb A1c levels compared with patients receiving usual care [11].

Planned care by a diabetes team at a Kaiser Permanente site was associated with a decrease in Hb A1c levels for patients with initially elevated levels in both the planned care and the usual care groups; blood pressures decreased in the planned care but not the usual care group. Hospital utilization decreased significantly over a 2-year period for patients who continued to receive planned care during the 2 years, but did not decrease for those who received planned care for only a short time. The hospital utilization finding suggests that to be successful, planned care needs to be sustained rather than episodic [12].

A Cochrane review summarized six controlled trials on the impact of care management by specialized nurses on short- and long-term clinical outcomes for patients with diabetes. Hb A1c levels were not significantly different between the planned care and the usual care groups over a

12-month period. The review concluded that care management may improve diabetic control over short time periods, but without ongoing care management improvements wane [13].

A Cochrane review, looking at seven studies of planned visits by nurses, found generally improved glycemic control and concluded that nurses "can even replace physicians in delivering many aspects of diabetes care, if detailed management protocols are available, or if they receive training"[14].

Of five studies involving diabetes *miniclinics*, which provided planned care in the primary care setting in the United Kingdom, four found improved outcomes [15]. One study of similar miniclinics in a U.S. integrated delivery system found that patients who attended the planned miniclinic visits had lower Hb A1c levels than patients receiving usual care [16]. This study is a reminder that some patients, accustomed to traditional physician visits, may *no-show* to planned visits, and that the effectiveness of planned visits depends on making them attractive and convenient to patients.

A review of 15 studies on care management for patients with diabetes found improvement of Hb A1c compared with controls, but no difference in lipid levels, blood pressures, or body mass index [17]. In another study, care management by a pharmacist resulted in significant improvement in Hb A1c levels compared with usual care [18].

Hypertension

A review of physician-nurse team approaches to blood pressure control found improvements in outcomes [19]. A review of 42 studies found that nursing participation in the care of people with hypertension promoted blood pressure reduction, weight loss, smoking cessation, increased physical activity, better medication adherence, and reduced physician visits [20].

Asthma

A review of pharmacist planned visits for patients with asthma found improved outcomes if the pharmacist had a detailed protocol, targeted patients with uncontrolled asthma, and worked in a practice system facilitating pharmacy care [21].

A randomized controlled trial of adults seen in the emergency department for asthma attacks found that patients offered three planned visits with specialized asthma nurses, compared with those receiving usual care, had higher peak flow measurements and fewer symptoms and acute attacks at 6 months of follow-up. The planned-care patients had fewer days off work at 3 months of follow-up, a finding that was not found at 6 months of follow-up. Planned nurse visits were effective, but the improvements were less evident over the long term, suggesting that planned care needs to be ongoing [22].

A Cochrane review of interventions for patients with adult asthma corroborated that regular practitioner review—sustained follow-up—is an important contributor to improved asthma outcomes [23].

A randomized controlled trial of nurse-led planned home visits for children with asthma-related hospital admissions found a significant reduction in asthma symptoms, readmissions, and urgent physician or emergency department visits for the planned-care group compared with a control group [24].

A randomized controlled trial of adults with asthma or chronic obstructive pulmonary disease found that those receiving planned visits by trained pharmacists had better peak flow rates than patients receiving usual care, but surprisingly, the planned visit patients had more emergency department visits than usual care patients [25].

Schulte found that care management improves outcomes in childhood asthma; success is due to care managers spending time working with families and building trusting relationships [26].

Congestive Heart Failure

Many studies have looked at interventions involving planned nurse visits—in the home, at a clinic, and/or by telephone—for patients discharged from the hospital for congestive heart failure (CHF). Some are referenced in Chapter 5. Overall, these interventions are highly successful in reducing rehospitalizations, indicating that the patients are less symptomatic from heart failure. Programs that include home visits are essential for success; telephone alone creates a lesser effect [27].

Coronary Heart Disease

Nurse-led planned care clinics for secondary prevention of coronary heart disease resulted in improved use of aspirin, better blood pressure and lipid management, and behavior change for exercise and diet (but not for smoking) compared with usual care. With a mean follow-up of 4.7 years, total adjusted mortality and coronary events appeared to be lower in the planned-care group [28].

A study of nurse-run care management to reduce coronary risk in patients following myocardial infarction found that the care-managed patients had greater rates of smoking cessation and lower LDL (low density lipoprotein)-cholesterol levels than patients receiving usual care [29].

Anticoagulation

Patients attending planned-care clinics for conditions requiring anticoagulation have fewer complications of anticoagulation treatment than patients whose anticoagulation is managed in routine primary care [30, 31].

Depression

A systematic review of disease management programs (using a variety of Chronic Care Model components) for patients with depression found that these programs showed significant improvement in processes and outcomes of care; precisely which Chronic Care Model components were effective is not clear [32].

Mixed Chronic Diseases

In a review of studies involving planned home visits by nurses to patients with a variety of chronic conditions, Frich found positive outcomes when many visits took place over a long period of time [33].

For more difficult patients, planned visits may fall short. Chronic care clinics for frail, elderly patients, including physician, nurse, and pharmacist visits, and a self-management/support group were held for a half day every 3–4 months. After 24 months, no significant improvements in incontinence, falls, depression, physical function, or prescriptions for high-risk medications were found compared with usual care, and costs of care were not different between the two groups. For complex problems, intensive care management and comprehensive practice change may be needed [34].

Six out of 6 studies of care management programs in primary care for patients with CHF, diabetes, and mixed comorbidities found improved outcomes compared with controls [35]. Intensive care management appears to be a successful system redesign, though it is expensive and generally reserved for patients at high risk.

CLINICAL INFORMATION SYSTEMS

Registries

A Cochrane review of five diabetes trials found that systems that identify patients at risk and bring those patients into care demonstrate slightly reduced Hb A1c levels compared with usual care [36]. A randomized trial of diabetes registries found that registries that generated *hot lists* of patients not in compliance with guidelines were significantly less successful in reducing Hb A1c levels for patients with initially high levels compared with registries that were also used to send reminder letters to patients [37]. This study underscores that by themselves, registries have no impact; they need to be used actively to intervene in care.

Clinician feedback

A Cochrane review looked at 85 studies on audit of physician performance on several clinical measures and feedback of these measures to physicians. Audit and feedback can be effective in improving professional practice, and the effect is larger when the baseline adherence to recommended practice is low [38]. Another review looking at physician feedback reported only 10 out of 24 studies showing positive results [2].

A review of 26 randomized controlled trials looked at provider reminders, feedback to providers, and combinations of reminders and feedback in improving physician medication management for a variety of conditions. A combination of feedback and reminders was no more effective than reminders alone. The authors concluded that reminders were more effective than feedback [39].

The patients of clinicians receiving *report cards* on their performance in the care of elderly patients did not improve their functional status or social support compared with patients of physicians not receiving report cards. In a meta-analysis of provider feedback for a variety of chronic conditions, 9 of 23 studies had positive results and there was an overall small but significant improvement in disease control [40].

Weiss and Wagner came to the conclusion that, while performance measurement and feedback of clinical measures to physicians has become a common practice, studies have not yet shown that this practice improves clinical care. Physician-specific feedback is problematic because of the need to risk-adjust the data, and because the number of patients with a specific condition seen by one physician is often insufficient to allow for a statistically meaningful comparison [41]. Feedback of performance data may be more useful for clinical sites rather than for individual physicians, but it is not known whether this variety of feedback is effective. As pay-for-performance systems grow, performance feedback becomes increasingly important [42].

Reminder prompts

Reminder systems may involve placing a sheet of paper in front of a chart, reminding the care team that preventive or chronic care actions are needed, or may be done through *pop-ups* on an electronic medical record. Twenty-two of twenty-six studies on physician reminders for a variety of chronic and preventive services found improvement in physician performance [2]. However, the overuse of reminders in an information-overloaded environment can be counterproductive. In one small study, 63% of physicians ignored the reminders [43]. Reminders may be most helpful when combined with team care, with a nonphysician team member acting on reminder prompts.

Looking at provider reminders for several chronic conditions, Weingarten and colleagues found a small but significant improvement, with the most effective programs targeting diabetes and hyperlipidemia [40]. Provider reminders to prescribe ACE (angiotensin-converting enzyme) inhibitors or statins in appropriate patients had little effect on increasing ACE inhibitor use but had no effect on statin use [44]. A review of interventions to increase the rate of cervical and breast cancer screening found that physician reminders were the most effective approach, resulting in a 40% increase in screening rates [45].

In a study conducted in Veterans Affairs (VA) clinics, computerized reminder prompts improved resident physicians' compliance with practice guidelines compared with a control group; however, the benefit of reminders declined over the 17-month course of the study suggesting that physicians develop a tendency to ignore the reminders [46].

Reminders can be sent to patients rather than targeted to physicians. Patient reminder systems' impact on childhood and adult immunization rates were positive in 33 of 41 studies of private practices, public health clinics, and academic settings. Telephone reminders were more effective than postcards or letters [47]. A meta-analysis evaluating patient reminders found a small but significant improvement [40]. An analysis of 46 interventions to increase cervical cancer screening concluded that mailed or telephone patient reminders were more effective than provider-targeted reminders. Reminders targeting both patients and providers were no more effective than reminders to patients or providers alone [48].

MULTIPLE CHRONIC CARE MODEL COMPONENT INTERVENTIONS

A review by Tsai and associates asked two questions: do interventions that incorporate at least one element of the Chronic Care Model result in improved chronic disease outcomes? Are any elements essential for improved outcomes? Looking at 112 studies on asthma, CHF, depression, and diabetes, the authors found that interventions with at least one Chronic Care Model element had consistently beneficial effects on clinical processes and outcomes across all four conditions. The most effective model elements were self-management support and delivery system design, and these were often bundled together with at least one other element. Decision support tended to improve processes of care but not outcomes. No single Chronic Care Model element was essential for improved outcomes. Data from studies with multiple Chronic Care Model elements did not support the notion that the elements are synergistic [49].

A systematic review of 24 studies examining a variety of Chronic Care Model components found a modest improvement in glycemic control for the diabetic patients in the intervention groups compared with controls. Of the five studies measuring systolic blood pressure control, only one reported a significant reduction for intervention group patients. One of three studies measuring LDL-cholesterol found that the intervention had a significant effect [50].

A Cochrane review on the management of obesity included 18 studies testing a variety of decision support, reminder system, and planned care interventions; the authors were unable to ascertain which intervention or combination of interventions is effective in improving patient behaviors or body mass index [51].

Hulscher and colleagues reviewed 55 studies on the delivery of preventive services in primary care. Physician reminders were consistently effective, and multifaceted interventions worked better than single interventions [52].

A study of decision support plus planned visits for patients with depression reduced the number of days with depression [53].

A Cochrane review of interventions to improve control of blood pressure examined 59 randomized controlled trials. Regular follow-up linked to vigorous drug therapy reduced blood pressure and all-cause mortality at 5 years follow-up. Appointment reminders improved rates of follow-up. Decision support for professionals did not have much of an effect, and planned visits seemed to be a promising innovation but need further evaluation [54].

A comparison of diabetes care quality within the VA system and commercial managed care organizations found that patients in the VA system had better control of LDL-cholesterol and Hb A1c, but not of blood pressure. The VA's superior results were related to a combination of Chronic Care Model components including a registry, provider feedback, patient reminders, and decision support [55].

A Cochrane review of studies on smoking cessation found that a combination of health professional training (decision support) and provider reminder systems increased the rate of professionals offering smoking cessation advice but had no impact on patient quit rates [56].

A Danish multiple-component intervention of 970 diabetic patients cared for by 474 general practitioners compared usual care with decision support, reminders, planned visits, and self-management training. After 6 years, Hb A1c, blood pressure, and lipids were significantly lower in the intervention group [57].

A review of 27 studies of mixed Chronic Care Model components for patients with diabetes found a significant improvement of Hb A1c for intervention group patients compared with controls, but no significant different in lipid levels, blood pressures, or body mass index [17].

REFERENCES

1. Cabana MD, Rand CS, Powe NR, et al: Why don't physicians follow clinical practice guidelines? JAMA. 1999;282:1458–1465.
2. Davis DA, Thomson MA, Oxman AD, et al: Changing physician performance. JAMA. 1995; 274:700–705.

3. Thomson O'Brien MA, Freemantle N, et al: Continuing education meetings and workshops: effects on professional practice and health care outcomes. Cochrane Database Syst Rev. 2005, Issue 3.
4. Thomson O'Brien MA, Oxman AD, et al: Educational outreach visits: effects on professional practice and health care outcomes. Cochrane Database Syst Rev. 2005, Issue 3.
5. Freemantle N, Harvey EL, Wolf F, et al: Printed educational materials: effects on professional practice and health care outcomes. Cochrane Database Syst Rev. 2000;(2):CD000172.
6. Tu K, Davis D: Can we alter physician behavior by educational methods? J Contin Educ Health Prof. 2002;22:11–22.
7. Kawamoto K, Houlihan CA, Balas A, et al: Improving clinical practice using decision support systems. BMJ. 2005;330:765–772.
8. Sadur CN, Moline N, Costa M, et al: Diabetes management in a health maintenance organization: efficacy of care management using cluster visits. Diabetes Care. 1999;22:2011–2017.
9. Peters AL, Davidson MB: Application of a diabetes managed care program. Diabetes Care. 1998;21:1037–1043.
10. Aubert RE, Herman WH, Waters J, et al: Nurse case management to improve glycemic control in diabetic patients in a health maintenance organization. Ann Intern Med. 1998;129:605–612.
11. Weinberger M, Kirkman MS, Samsa GP: A nurse-coordinated intervention for primary care patients with non–insulin–dependent diabetes mellitus. J Gen Intern Med. 1995;10:59–66.
12. Domurat ES: Diabetes managed care and clinical outcomes. Am J Manag Care. 1999;5:1299–1307.
13. Loveman E, Royle P, Waugh N: Specialist nurses in diabetes mellitus. Cochrane Database Syst Rev. 2005, Issue 3.
14. Renders CM, Valk GD, Griffin S, et al: Interventions to improve the management of diabetes mellitus in primary care, outpatient, and community settings. Cochrane Database Syst Rev. 2005, Issue 3.
15. Farmer A, Coulter A: Organization of care for diabetic patients in general practice. Br J Gen Pract. 1990;40:56–58.
16. Wagner EH, Grothaus LC, Sandhu N, et al: Chronic care clinics for diabetes in primary care: a system-wide randomized trial. Diabetes Care. 2001;24:695–700.
17. Norris SL, Nichols PJ, Caspersen CJ, et al: The effectiveness of disease and case management for people with diabetes. Am J Prev Med. 2002;22(4S):15–38.
18. Choe HM, Mitrovich S, Dubay D, et al: Proactive case management of high-risk patients with type 2 diabetes mellitus by a clinical pharmacist. Am J Manag Care. 2005;11:253–260.

19. Norby SM, Stroebel RJ, Canzanello VJ: Physician-nurse team approaches to improve blood pressure control. J Clin Hypertens. 2003;5:386–392.

20. Bengtson A, Dreverhorn E: The nurse's role and skills in hypertension care: a review. Clin Nurse Spec. 2003;17:260–268.

21. McLean WM, MacKeigan LD: When does pharmaceutical care impact health outcomes? A comparison of community pharmacy-based studies of pharmaceutical care for patients with asthma. Ann Pharmacother. 2005;39:625–631.

22. Levy ML, Robb M, Allen J, et al: A randomized controlled evaluation of specialist nurse education following accident and emergency department attendance for acute asthma. Respir Med. 2000;94:900–908.

23. Gibson PG, Powell H, Coughlan J, et al: Self-management education and regular practitioner review for adults with asthma. Cochrane Database Syst Rev. 2005, Issue 3.

24. Madge P, McColl J, Paton J: Impact of a nurse-led home management training programme in children admitted to hospital with acute asthma. Thorax. 1997;52:223–228.

25. Weinberger M, Murray MD, Marrero DG, et al: Effectiveness of pharmacist care for patients with reactive airways disease. JAMA. 2002;288: 1594–1602.

26. Schulte A, Musolf J, Meurer JR, et al: Pediatric asthma case management. J Pediatr Nurs. 2004;19:304–310.

27. Wagner EH: Deconstructing heart failure disease management. Ann Intern Med. 2004;131:644–646.

28. Murchie P, Campbell NC, Ritchie LD, et al: Nurse-led clinics for the secondary prevention of coronary heart disease. BMJ. 2003;326:84–87.

29. DeBusk RF, Miller NH, Superko R, et al: A case-management system for coronary risk factor modification after acute myocardial infarction. Ann Intern Med. 1994;120:721–729.

30. Hamby L, Weeks WB, Malikowski C: Complications of warfarin therapy: causes, costs, and the role of the anticoagulation clinic. Eff Clin Pract. 2000;4:179–184.

31. Chiquette E, Amato MG, Bussey HI: Comparison of an anti-coagulation clinic with usual medical care. Arch Intern Med. 1998;158:1641–1647.

32. Badamgarav E, Weingarten SR, Henning JM, et al: Effectiveness of disease management programs in depression: a systematic review. Am J Psychiatry. 2003;160:2080–2090.

33. Frich LM: Nursing interventions for patients with chronic conditions. J Adv Nurs. 2003;44:137–153.

34. Coleman EA, Grothaus LC, Sandhu N, et al: Chronic care clinics: a randomized controlled trial of a new model of primary care for frail older adults. J Am Geriatr Soc. 1999;47:775–783.

35. Ferguson JA, Weinberger M: Case management programs in primary care. J Gen Intern Med. 1998;13:123–126.
36. Griffin S, Kinmonth AL: Systems for routine surveillance for people with diabetes mellitus. Cochrane Database Syst Rev. 2005, Issue 3.
37. Stroebel RJ, Scheitel SM, Fitz JS, et al: A randomized trial of three diabetes registry implementation strategies in a community internal medicine practice. Jt Comm J Qual Improv. 2002;28:441–450.
38. Jamtvedt G, Young JM, Kristoffersen DT, et al: Audit and feedback: effects on professional practice and health care outcomes. Cochrane Database of Syst Rev. 2005, Issue 3.
39. Bennett JW, Glasziou PP: Computerized reminders and feedback in medication management. Med J Aust. 2003;178:217–222.
40. Weingarten SR, Henning JM, Badamgarav E, et al: Interventions used in disease management programmes for patients with chronic illness—which ones work? BMJ. 2002;325:925–933.
41. Weiss KB, Wagner R: Performance measurement through audit, feedback and profiling as tools for improving chronic care. Chest. 2000;118(Suppl): 53S-58S.
42. Epstein AM, Lee TH, Hamel MB: Paying physicians for high-quality care. N Engl J Med. 2004;350:406–410.
43. Lawson K: Electronic reminders can get lost in info overload. Internal Medicine News, August 1, 2000, p. 34.
44. Derose SF, Dudl JR, Benson VM, et al: Point-of-service reminders for prescribing cardiovascular medicines. Am J Manag Care. 2005;11:298–304.
45. Kupets R, Covens A: Strategies for the implementation of cervical and breast cancer screening of women by primary care physicians. Gynecol Oncol. 2001;83:186–197.
46. Demakis JG, Beauchamp C, Cull WL, et al: Improving residents' compliance with standards of ambulatory care. JAMA. 2000;284:1411–1416.
47. Szilagyi PG, Bordley C, Vann JC, et al: Effect of patient reminder/recall interventions on immunization rates. JAMA. 2000;284:1820–1827.
48. Yabroff KR, Mangan P, Mandelblatt J: Effectiveness of interventions to increase Papanicolaou smear use. J Am Board Fam Pract. 2003;16: 188–203.
49. Tsai AC, Morton SC, Mangione CM, et al: A meta-analysis of interventions to improve care for chronic illness. Am J Manag Care. 2005;11:478–488.
50. Knight K, Badamgarav E, Henning JM, et al: A systematic review of diabetes disease management programs. Am J Managed Care 2005;11: 242–250.
51. Harvey EL, Glenny A-M, Kirk SFL, et al: Improving health professionals' management and the organization of care for overweight and obese people. Cochrane Database Syst Rev. 2005, Issue 3.

52. Hulscher ME, Wensing M, van Der Weijden T, et al: Interventions to implement prevention in primary care. Cochrane Database Syst Rev. 2001;(1): CD000362.
53. Schoenbaum M, Unutzer J, Sherbourne C, et al: Cost-effectiveness of practice-initiated quality improvement for depression. JAMA. 2001;286: 1325–1330.
54. Fahey T, Schroeder K, Ebrahim S: Interventions used to improve control of blood pressure in patients with hypertension. Cochrane Database Syst Rev. 2005, Issue 3.
55. Kerr EA, Gerzoff RB, Krein SL, et al: Diabetes care quality in the Veterans Affairs health care system and commercial managed care: the TRIAD study. Ann Intern Med. 2004;141:272–281.
56. Lancaster T, Silagy C, Fowler G: Training health professionals in smoking cessation. Cochrane Database Syst Rev. 2005, Issue 3.
57. Olivarius NF, Beck-Nielsen H, Andreasen AH, et al: Randomised controlled trial of structured personal care of type 2 diabetes mellitus. BMJ. 2001;323:970–975.

Review of Evidence on Primary Care Teams

While studies of team models are difficult to perform [1], the research presented here provides important insights into team care.

FACTORS ASSOCIATED WITH WELL-FUNCTIONING TEAMS

A research group in the United Kingdom produced a 400-page report, *The Effectiveness of Health Care Teams in the National Health Service* [2]. The researchers gathered information from 100 randomly selected primary health care teams, 113 community mental health care teams, and 193 secondary health care teams.

Team cohesion was assessed with the degree of participation of team members, the clarity of objectives, an emphasis on quality, the striving for innovation, and the use of team problem solving. The outcomes measured, which the authors called *team effectiveness*, included 21 parameters in the areas of teamwork, patient satisfaction and clinical outcomes, and organizational efficiency. Some of the patient measures were immunization rates, other health promotion activities, use of evidence-based management of chronic diseases, numbers of hospital admissions, waiting times for appointments, and ease of telephone access. Team member stress and turnover were measured.

Numerous studies in non–health care environments have shown the importance of leadership in creating effective teams. Primary care team members in England rated their effectiveness more highly when they had strong leadership and high involvement of all team members [3]. Effective decision-making processes are central to team performance. A dilemma that teams need to solve is that participatory decision making increases job satisfaction; yet team members with more clinical training (physicians) in fact make, and possibly should make, most of the decisions [2].

Establishing guidelines and processes by which team members communicate is necessary; haphazard communication can be destructive. Large-size teams experience great strains on effective communication. When teams exceed 12 members, they have difficulties [2]. Moreover, larger team size reduces continuity of care and patient access to their personal clinician [4].

Team functioning can be enhanced through selection of skilled and motivated team members, team-building interventions, setting clear and agreed-upon goals, and obtaining feedback on progress toward goal achievement. Effective teams engage in problem solving to improve team functioning [2].

Race and gender have an impact on team functioning. In one study, racially diverse team members evaluated team communication according to different perspectives and alternative realities. Stereotyping served to reinforce these differences and deepen communication problems [5]. Gender considerations are also important; in primary care teams, women dominate in number but men predominate in the high-status positions [6].

Not only are intrateam processes important determinants of team effectiveness; the support of the team by the larger organization influences team effectiveness powerfully. Teams receiving no rewards, no feedback, no clear objectives, inadequate working conditions, and ineffective relationships with other teams are less likely to function well [2]. Reward systems, such as public recognition, preferred work assignments, and money, enhance motivation and performance. Team performance is most effective when rewards are administered to the team as a whole and not to individuals [7]. Team formation is easier in larger practices and takes place only when payment systems reward team development [4].

External feedback to teams helps to confirm realistic goals and foster team commitment. Training and technical assistance in team functioning are needed for successful team performance. Teams sharing the same physical space are more effective than teams dispersed across sites [2].

The Canadian Health Transition Fund was an experiment in primary care team formation that came to similar conclusions as the UK study. The success of team building depended on: (1) interpersonal relations between team members, (2) conditions within the health care organization, and (3) larger society values. Important determinants of successful team building included: overcoming unequal power relations, differing values, and strong professional (rather than patient-centered) identification that creates tensions between physicians and other professionals; creating a climate within the health care organization that fosters physical proximity of team members, time to conduct group discussions, realistic objectives, clear division of work, the formalization of rules and procedures for team functioning, and administrative support for interprofessional collaboration; and building trust among the team members. The Canadian experiment conquered some barriers to team formation but was unable to overcome others [8].

These studies suggest that health care organizations desiring to reorganize care into teams often fail to understand the energy required to initiate and sustain teams. Well-functioning teams are those that have created protocols defining division of labor among team members, required all team members to be trained in the tasks within their job descriptions, and set aside time for team meetings. Because these team-building efforts increase costs and may reduce revenues, organizations may not choose to make the necessary investment in team development, resulting in team failure.

ARE WELL-FUNCTIONING TEAMS ASSOCIATED WITH BETTER OUTCOMES THAN POORLY FUNCTIONING TEAMS OR NO TEAMS?

Campbell et al. studied a stratified random sample of 60 general practices in six areas of England, examining the quality of chronic and preventive care, access to care, continuity of care, and patient satisfaction. Many clinical outcomes and results of patient surveys to 200 randomly selected patients from each practice were associated with practice characteristics, including team climate, which were measured from questionnaires from staff members employed by the practices. Team climate was measured as a composite score from staff perceptions of how people work together, how frequently they interact, whether teams have identified aims and objectives, and how much practical support is given toward improved ways of doing things. Scores for diabetes care, overall patient satisfaction, and patient assessment of continuity of care, and access to care were significantly higher in practices with higher scores on team climate. Clinical quality for asthma, coronary heart disease, and preventive services were not significantly associated with team climate. Another practice characteristic strongly associated with improved chronic care was the length of the physician visit [9].

Stevenson et al. asked what features of primary health care teams were associated with quality improvement of diabetes care. Forty-three primary care teams in the United Kingdom were fed data on six diabetes process measures; each team met to agree on an action plan to improve its performance and data collection was repeated in 12 months. The mean of the improvement for the six measures was calculated at baseline and 12 months. Improvement scores varied between 44% for one practice and minus 13% for the least successful practice. Separate interviews were conducted with two members of the nine teams that had improved the most and the nine that had improved the least. Positive perceptions of how the team functioned were correlated with improved diabetes scores. Teams that reported disharmony had lower scores [10].

Jansson and colleagues analyzed the records of general practitioners and district caregivers over 6 years in Sweden. Care teams—GP (general practitioner), district nurse, assistant nurse—were introduced into one region but were absent in another comparative region. The care teams reported a large rise in the overall number of patient contacts and in the proportion of the population who accessed the district nurse. Concurrently, there was a reduction in emergency visits [11].

In the United States, Eggert and colleagues demonstrated that a team-driven case management system for elderly patients reduced total health care expenditures by 13.6% when compared to an individualized case management system. The team combined earlier discharge, more timely nursing home placement, and better-organized home support to reduce patient hospitalization by 26% [12].

Jones reported that families who received team care had fewer hospitalizations, fewer operations, less physician visits for illness, and more physician visits for health supervision than control families [13].

Goni studied primary care teams in a region of Spain in which each team is responsible for a panel of patients residing in a defined geographic area; 256 physicians, nurses, and other caregivers working in 31 teams were surveyed regarding team functioning; and the regional governmental authority overseeing primary care provided data on team efficiency (number of consultations per health care personnel) and patient satisfaction. Team functioning was measured by respondents' answers to the survey regarding the clarity of team goals, empowerment of team members to participate fully, cooperative relationships among team members, clear delineation of tasks, and team members feeling appreciated for their work. Nineteen of the teams were classified as high functioning and twelve as low functioning. The high-functioning teams were associated with greater patient satisfaction, but not with increased efficiency [14].

Roblin and colleagues studied 25 primary care teams in the Georgia region of Kaiser Permanente's large integrated delivery system. The research group created a measure of team functioning, called the cooperative clinical culture (CCC), including such variables as delegation of tasks, collaboration, patient familiarity, time to perform tasks, and the ability of the team to make its own decisions within the larger organization. The CCC of each team was judged by a written survey of team members. Outcomes included patient satisfaction, average Hb A1c and LDL—cholesterol of patients with diabetes, use of inhaled steroids for patients with persistent asthma. Initial findings showed that teams with higher CCC scores were associated with greater patient satisfaction and better chronic disease quality for patients with diabetes and asthma [15].

The *Effectiveness of Health Care Teams* study is the largest research effort attempting to demonstrate an association between team functioning and team outcomes. The study used multiple regression analysis to identify which team attributes were associated with better or worse outcomes. The outcomes were based on internal ratings of team performance by team members and external ratings of team performance by regional health authorities. With one exception—hospital mortality—outcomes did not include measures of objective clinical quality or surveys of patient satisfaction. The study concluded that the quality of team performance is powerfully related to the clarity of team objectives, the level of participation and commitment to quality by team members, and the degree of support for innovation. The percentage of hospital staff working in teams was found to be inversely associated with hospital mortality. Well-functioning teams had less staff turnover than poorly functioning teams. Communication and regular meetings in primary care teams were associated with higher levels of performance, though the quality of team meetings in primary care was often poor. Teams with unclear leadership had lower levels of staff participation, commitment to quality, and staff satisfaction. Conflict over leadership was found to be disastrous for teams [2].

WHO SHOULD BE THE PLAYERS ON THE PRIMARY CARE TEAM?

Composition of primary care teams varies greatly depending on the type of practice, from the solo practitioner's office with one person tending to front office, back office, and billing functions to the large hospital outpatient clinic or multispecialty practice. Rural versus urban settings [16] and offices close to versus far away from hospitals influence the availability of personnel. Experiments are taking place in the United States and Canada to organize dispersed teams, with personnel in different locations. communicating by e-mail, telephone, and occasional meetings about the care of a group of patients [17, 18].

Choosing personnel for a primary care team is based on three motivations: the skill mix needed to enhance clinical quality, the substitution of less costly nonphysician labor for more highly paid physicians, and the importance of preserving continuity of care in an era of increasingly part-time physicians.

Skill mix

Team members may contribute unique talents that enhance the quality of the practice. Wagner has argued that nurses' training makes them better than physicians at following chronic care management protocols. Nurse practitioners may also have better patient education and communication skills than physicians [19]. In a U.S. teaching hospital, a comparison of patients with diabetes and hypertension randomly assigned to a physician-nurse practitioner team versus a physician alone found costs to be higher for the team; however, team patients had significant improvements in Hb A1c, HDL-cholesterol, and satisfaction with care compared with non-team patients [20].

Sommers and colleagues compared primary care teams with physician-only care across 18 private practices, concluding that team practices lowered hospitalization rates and reduced physician visits while maintaining function for elderly patients with chronic illness and functional deficits. Cost savings from reduced hospitalization accounted for more than the costs of setting up the team and making regular home visits. Increased satisfaction by patients receiving team care, compared with those receiving physician-only care, appeared to be related to more social activities, fewer symptoms, and slightly improved overall health [21].

Other studies suggest that multidisciplinary clinical teams produce clinical outcomes superior to those achieved by usual care arrangements, with many of these studies evaluating the addition of nurses, social workers, psychologists, and clinical pharmacists to teams [22, 23].

The creation of teams with personnel from several disciplines may be the fundamental primary care redesign that allows other components of the Chronic Care Model to succeed (see Chapter 4). Team care allows delegation by the physician of chronic care responsibilities to other team members. Appendix N demonstrates evidence that the addition of care managers—nurses, pharmacists [24–26], or (in the case of asthma) respiratory therapists—makes planned chronic care visits possible and allows patient self-management support (see Chapter 5) to take place.

Substitution

Another motivation for adding team members is to conserve expensive physician labor through substitution of other personnel for physician effort. Studies of substitution by nonphysician clinicians are reviewed in Chapter 9.

Continuity of care

With primary care physicians tending to work fewer hours per week, the challenges of providing continuity of care mount. The creation of teams— for example, a physician-nurse practitioner team or a half-time physician dyad—with at least one team member available during all practice hours can reduce fragmentation of care for patients.

Surprisingly, Parkerton and colleagues found that part-time physicians, compared with physicians working longer hours, achieved slightly higher rates of cancer screening and diabetes management process measures; there was no association of patient satisfaction with the number of physician hours worked per week [27].

The same research group studied the association between continuity of care, practice coordination, and those same clinical outcomes (cancer screening, diabetes management, and patient satisfaction). Practice coordination involved two surrogates of *teamness*: shared practice (two or three physicians who shared responsibility for a panel of patients) and team tenure (the number of years that physicians in a primary care site had worked with one another). On average, only 42% of visits within one year were between a patient and the patient's designated primary care physician. Yet increased continuity of care was not associated with improved measures for any of the three outcomes. In contrast, the two teamness measures—shared practices and team tenure—were associated with improved cancer screening and diabetes management. Team tenure was also associated with patient satisfaction [28]. These studies suggest that practices functioning as teams of physicians and nurse practitioners can perform as well as full-time physicians who offer continuity of care to their patients.

HOW DO PRIMARY CARE TEAMS FUNCTION IN THE REAL WORLD?

Several studies have observed teams in primary care. Based on their experience from the Martin Luther King health center in the South Bronx in the 1960s, Harold Wise and colleagues wrote *Making Health Teams Work*, a book rich in anecdotes and lessons. Frustrated with the difficulties of getting humans to work together, Dr. Wise at one point asserts that the ideal size of a health care team is one person [29]. The difficulties of melding a health care team are echoed by Banta and Fox in their description of the stresses and strains felt by the primary care team at Columbia Point Health Center in Boston [30].

Shaw interviewed GPs, managers, and nurses in 21 primary care practices in low-income areas of London regarding the functioning of their clinical teams. Due to the deprivation of the patients, the practices tended to be highly stressed, making it difficult to attract and retain personnel. A number of the physicians dominated the practice and did not allow other professionals to make significant decisions. Most respondents judged teamworking to be poor; personnel turnover made teamwork impossible [31].

Patel et al., studying a primary care team at a U.S. teaching hospital, had a more positive message. The team included three faculty physicians, a psychiatrist, two medical residents, two nurse practitioners, a clinical nurse, a social worker, an HIV (human immunodeficiency virus) case manager, a community resource specialist, and two administrators. Team members had demarcated tasks and areas of responsibility, but with considerable overlap. A component of successful interactions was the hierarchical structure based on the degree of expertise of each team member. Most communication among team members was done face-to-face and was related to the clinical problems of the team's patients. While face-to-face communication was productive 99–100% of the time, telephone communication failed 20% of the time due to the telephone not being available. Physical proximity of team members greatly enhanced communication. The authors concluded that while successful collaboration among team members is helpful, quality of care is chiefly based on the knowledge and expertise of each team member [32].

Cashman et al. studied team development at a U.S. community health center from 1999 to 2001. The health center was organized into three teams, each including a physician, nurse practitioner, physician assistant, registered nurse, outreach worker, and medical assistant. One team attended five training workshops over a 2-year period and held 3 hours of team meetings per month. During the training process, team members expressed greater cooperation with one another, increased knowledge of each member's roles and responsibilities, and greater appreciation for the strengths of their colleagues. However, by the end of the study period, the team climate had deteriorated back to baseline as team members were frustrated by difficulties in making clinical improvements and by the problem of turnover—valuable team members leaving the organization. The authors summarized the barriers to team cohesion: heterogeneity of team composition, role conflict and role overload, and constraints placed on the team by the larger organization. Without support of the larger organization, teams could not be effective [33].

Charles-Jones and colleagues studied the redistribution of primary care tasks in the United Kingdom, with the evolution from an autonomous physician structure to a greater team orientation. These changes have in part been stimulated by governmental demands that primary care improve timely access to care and the quality of chronic disease care. These dual pressures have forced general practitioners to delegate clinical work to nurses and health care assistants. The emergence of primary care teams has increased the complexity of the primary care enterprise, with triage nurses judging which patients need to see which caregivers [34]. The authors interviewed GPs, nurses, and practice managers from nine practices, looking at the issue of triage as a key determinant of how tasks are allocated in the team. Some physicians were happy with the delegation of minor ailments to nurses while others felt that the physician should handle all patient complaints. Some nurses enjoyed becoming more of a diagnostician while others were unhappy that they were not following physician orders to change dressings and perform other hands-on functions. A number of physicians, nurses, and managers felt that the team-based system was more efficient, but less patient centered since the patients were not allowed to choose which team member they were channeled to see. Others, particularly nurses, felt that patients felt more comfortable seeing the nurse than the physician [34].

The Effectiveness of Health Care Teams study, observing 100 primary care practices, reported that meetings in primary care sites were often poorly managed and dysfunctional. Meetings were frequently cancelled or started late. When the teams did meet, many team members did not participate. In over half the meetings studied, no group decisions were made. In spite of all these problems, improved meeting attendance was associated with better care. The study also found that leadership, an essential factor for successful teams, was often absent. Although effective teams engaged in problem-solving, some teams denied, distorted, or hid problems [2].

In another study, investigators interviewed 96 members of UK primary care teams. They highlighted the failure of teams to set aside time for regular meetings to define objectives, clarify roles, apportion tasks, and encourage participation. Poor communication was attributed to differences in status, power, educational background, and the assumption that doctors would be the leaders [35, 36].

Bond and colleagues surveyed about 300 general practitioner/nurse teams in the United Kingdom; they reported low levels of communication and collaboration between GPs and nursing staff [37]. Two other studies reached similar conclusions [38, 39].

For teams to function, patients must be willing to receive care from nonphysician team members. Sibbald et al. cite a number of studies showing that patients are satisfied with care provided by nurses for minor concerns but prefer physicians for serious problems [4].

REFERENCES

1. Schmitt MH, Farrell MP, Heinemann GD: Conceptual and methodologic problems in studying the effects of interdisciplinary geriatric teams. Gerontologist. 1988;28:753–764.
2. Borrill CS, Carletta J, Carter AJ, et al: *The Effectiveness of Health Care Teams in the National Health Service*. Birmingham, UK: Aston Centre for Health Service Organization Research, 2001.
3. Ross F, Rink E, Furne A: Integration or pragmatic coalition? An evaluation of nursing teams in primary care. J Interprof Care. 2000;14:259–267.
4. Sibbald B, Laurant M, Scott T: Changing task profiles. In Saltman R, Rico A, Boerma W (eds.): *Primary care in the Driver's Seat? Organizational Reform in European Primary Care*. Berkshire, UK, Open University Press, 2005.
5. Dreachslin JL, Hunt PL, Sprainer E: Workforce diversity: implications for the effectiveness of health care delivery teams. Social Sci Med. 2000;50: 1403–1414.
6. Jackson LA, Sullivan LA, Hodge LN: Stereotype effects on attributions, predictions, and evaluations. J Pers Soc Psychol. 1993;65:69–84.
7. Hackman JR (ed.): *Groups That Work (and Those That Don't): Creating Conditions for Effective Teamwork*. San Francisco, CA, Jossey-Bass, 1990.
8. San Martin-Rodriguez L, Beaulieu M-D, D'Amour D, et al: The determinants of successful collaboration. J Interprof Care. 2005;(Suppl 1): 132–147.
9. Campbell SM, Hann M, Hacker J, et al: Identifying predictors of high quality care in English general practice. BMJ. 2001;323:1–6.
10. Stevenson K, Baker R, Farooqi A, et al: Features of primary health care teams associated with successful quality improvement of diabetes care. Fam Pract. 2001;18:21–26.
11. Jansson A, Isacsson A, Lindhom LH: Organization of health care teams and the population's contacts with primary care. Scand J Health Care. 1992;10:257–265.
12. Eggert GM, Zimmer JG, Hall WJ: Case management: a randomised controlled study comparing a neighbourhood team and a centralized individual model. Health Serv Res. 1991;26:471–507.
13. Jones RVH: Teamworking in primary care: how do we know about it? J Interprof Care. 1992;6:25–29.
14. Goni S: An analysis of the effectiveness of Spanish primary care teams. Health Policy. 1999;48:107–117.
15. Roblin DW, Kaplan SH, Greenfield S, et al: Collaborative clinical culture and primary care outcomes. In: Program and abstracts of the annual meeting

of the Academy for Health Services Research and Quality, Washington, DC, June 23–25, 2002.

16. Farmer J, West C, Whyte B, et al: Primary health care teams as adaptive organizations. Health Serv Manage Res. 2005;18:151–164.

17. Farris KB, Cote I, Feeny D, et al: Enhancing primary care for complex patients. Can Fam Physician. 2004;50:998–1003.

18. Rothschild SK, Lapidos S, Minnick A, et al: Using virtual teams to improve the care of chronically ill patients. JCOM. 2004;11:346–350.

19. Wagner EH: The role of patient care teams in chronic disease management. BMJ. 2000;320:569–572.

20. Litaker D, Mion LC, Planavsky L, et al: Physician-nurse practitioner teams in chronic disease management. J Interprof Care. 2003;17:223–237.

21. Sommers LS, Marton KI, Barbaccia JC, et al: Physician, nurse, and social worker collaboration in primary care for chronically ill seniors. Arch Intern Med. 2000;160:1825–1833.

22. Wagner EH, Glasgow RE, Davis C, et al: Quality improvement in chronic illness care: a collaborative approach. Jt Comm J Qual Improv. 2001; 27:63–80.

23. Halstead LS: Team care in chronic illness: a critical review of the literature of the past 25 years. Arch Phys Med Rehabil. 1976;57:507–511.

24. Hanlon JT, Weinberger M, Samsa GP, et al: A randomized controlled trial of a clinical pharmacist intervention to improve inappropriate prescribing in elderly outpatients with polypharmacy. Am J Med. 1996;100:428–437.

25. Bogden PE, Abbott RD, Williamson P, et al: Comparing standard care with a physician and pharmacist team approach for uncontrolled hypertension. J Gen Intern Med. 1998;13:740–745.

26. Gattis WA, Hasselblad V, Whellan DJ, et al: Reduction in heart failure events by the addition of a clinical pharmacist to the heart failure team. Arch Intern Med. 1999;159:1939–1945.

27. Parkerton PH, Wagner EH, Smith DG, et al: Effect of part-time practice on patient outcomes. J Gen Intern Med. 2003;18:717–724.

28. Parkerton PH, Smith DG, Straley HL: Primary care practice coordination versus physician continuity. Fam Med. 2004;36:15–21.

29. Wise H, Beckhard R, Rubin I, et al: *Making Health Teams Work*. Cambridge, MA, Ballinger Publishing Co, 1974.

30. Banta HD, Fox RC: Role strains of a health care team in a poverty community. Soc Sci Med. 1972;6:697–722.

31. Shaw A, de Lusignan S, Rowlands G: Do primary care professionals work as a team: a qualitative study. J Interprof Care. 2005;19:396–405.

32. Patel VL, Cytryn KN, Shortliffe EH, et al: The collaborative health care team: the role of individual and group expertise. Teach Learn Med. 2000;12:117–132.

33. Cashman SB, Reidy P, Cody K, et al: Developing and measuring progress toward collaborative, integrated, interdisciplinary health care teams. J Interprof Care. 2004;18:183–196.
34. Charles-Jones H, Latimer J, May C: Transforming general practice: the redistribution of medical work in primary care. Sociol Health Illn. 2003;25: 71–92.
35. West MA, Field R: Teamwork in primary health care: perspectives from organisational psychology. J Interprof Care. 1995;9:117–122.
36. Field R, West MA: Teamwork in primary health care: two perspectives from practices. J Interprof Care. 1995;9:123–130.
37. Bond J, Cartilidge AM, Gregson BA, et al: A Study of Interprofessional Collaboration in Primary Health Care Organizations. Health Care Research Unit, University of Newcastle-upon-Tyne, 1985.
38. McClure LM: Teamwork, myth or reality: community nurses effectiveness with general practice attachment. J Epidemiol Community Health. 1984; 21:68–74.
39. Cant S, Killoran A: Team tactics: a study of nurse collaboration in general practice. Health Educ J. 1995;52:203–208.

Index

Page numbers followed by *f* or *t* indicate figures or tables, respectively.